P9-DME-345

Silver Linings:
The Other Side of Cancer

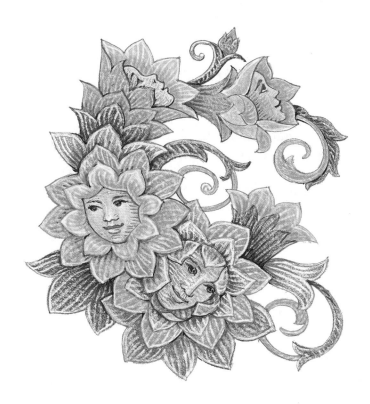

edited by
Shirley M. Gullo, RN, MSN, OCN® and
Elaine Glass, RN, MS, OCN®
with illustrations by Maria Gamiere

Oncology Nursing Press, Inc.
Pittsburgh, Pennsylvania

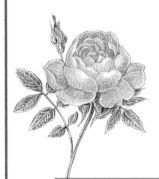

Library of Congress Card Catalog Number: 97-66193

ISBN 1-890504-01-7

Printed in the United States of America.

Oncology Nursing Press, Inc.
A Subsidiary of the Oncology Nursing Society

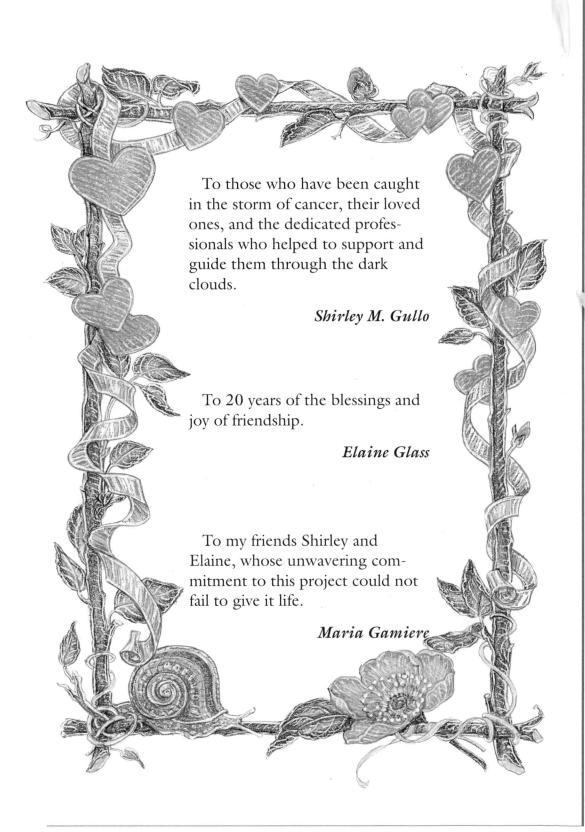

To those who have been caught in the storm of cancer, their loved ones, and the dedicated professionals who helped to support and guide them through the dark clouds.

Shirley M. Gullo

To 20 years of the blessings and joy of friendship.

Elaine Glass

To my friends Shirley and Elaine, whose unwavering commitment to this project could not fail to give it life.

Maria Gamiere

Contents

Preface

This book represents two important firsts for the Oncology Nursing Society. First, it is a book that gives our members the chance to share the stories they have heard and experiences they have had with their patients. These nurses have cried and laughed, but along the way, they have grown as people and nurses. Their stories are the answer to the often-asked question, "How can you take care of people with cancer? Isn't it too sad?" It also gives patients and their families an opportunity to share their feelings on the cancer experience, which can help both other patients and care providers understand the human side of this disease.

Silver Linings: The Other Side of Cancer also is the first book published by the Oncology Nursing Press, Inc. I hope that the authors and editors of this book have found working with the Oncology Nursing Press, Inc. staff another growing experience. Congratulations to all who made this book possible— patients, families, editors, authors, and the Oncology Nursing Press, Inc. staff.

Pearl Moore, RN, MN, FAAN
Executive Director, Oncology Nursing Society

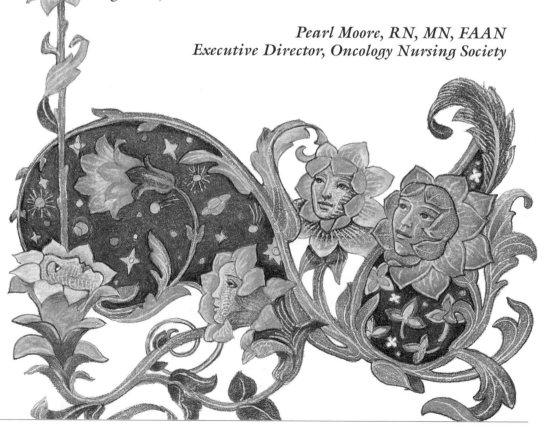

If you are reading this preface, you likely are confronting cancer either personally or as a loved one, friend, or healthcare provider. The cold, hard statistics of cancer say that it is a common disease, striking more than 1.3 million men, women, and children in the United States every year. Given these statistics, few of us will complete our life's journey without knowing cancer personally or as a family member of someone stricken by the disease. In whatever context, cancer irrevocably changes your life. Regardless of the prognosis, to know cancer is to come face to face with uncertainty. Assumptions about a long and uncomplicated life are suddenly shattered. Most find their world turned upside down.

At first it may be hard to believe that any good or positive experiences could come from having cancer. Yet even in the most difficult of circumstances, the human spirit prevails. Stripped to essentials, cancer helps each of us examine our priorities and reconnect with what is meaningful. Life becomes precious, and time becomes cherished in ways it never was before.

The greatest reward of being a cancer nurse is sharing the challenges of cancer and seeing the renewal of the human spirit in those for whom we care. Shirley Gullo and Elaine Glass have seen the silver linings of cancer. In conceiving of this project, they knew that we would draw strength and new perspectives from the stories of those experiencing cancer. These are stories that help and heal. They teach us how to live our lives with or without cancer, and they will challenge you to see the silver linings of your experience with cancer. As much as you need medical information before beginning treatment for cancer, you and your loved ones need the stories included in *Silver Linings: The Other Side of Cancer*. Healthcare providers will help you with the treatment of your disease, but these stories will help you reclaim the purpose and direction of your life as you continue your journey.

Kathi H. Mooney, RN, PhD, FAAN, AOCN
Past President, Oncology Nursing Society

Foreword

Life's garden takes preparation, planting, cultivating, and harvesting. Each of us has a personal investment in growing and learning from the obstacles we confront in life. A diagnosis of cancer is one of life's most challenging obstacles. Initially, the thought of growing or learning anything positive from the experience of cancer may seem ludicrous. However, the personal, true stories in *Silver Linings: The Other Side of Cancer* may change your mind and will surely touch your heart.

Successfully learning to walk begins with the first step. I strongly suggest that your first step be reading one story. It will probably take you less than five minutes. The stories are brief, easy to read, and meaningful. Each one has a unique message. It may address the author's struggle, a new love, closer relationships with family, a unique bond with new friends, an amusing incident, a new appreciation for the preciousness of life, or a spiritual awakening. One patient declared, "Cancer was a wake-up call!"

In their stories, people with cancer, their loved ones, friends, and nurses share their personal views as they traveled through the cancer experience. They describe the remarkable lessons they learned along the way, which resulted in a more beautiful life garden and a harvest they never thought possible.

As the husband of one who has journeyed through cancer, I encourage you to keep this beautifully illustrated book on your coffee table or nightstand. Pick it up every once in awhile for an insightful walk into the garden that others have planted and cultivated as a result of their experiences with cancer. I sincerely hope that your harvest from reading this book will be bountiful.

Leonard J. Staysniak
Husband of Anna, a cancer survivor
Ohio

Acknowledgments

This book has been a labor of love strengthened by the spirit of many. We preceded each step with prayer for guidance, wisdom, and strength. The book involved contributions from many people. We sincerely thank all of them for their essential contributions.

We gratefully acknowledge our oncology nursing colleagues who agreed that the project was worth pursuing and supported our book proposal. The encouragement of Pearl Moore, RN, MN, FAAN, executive director of the Oncology Nursing Society (ONS), provided additional confirmation that we were on the right path. Leonard Mafrica, deputy executive director of the Oncology Nursing Press, Inc., and his dedicated staff were our guides along the way.

Jan Kinzler, marketing and public relations team leader, began the process of soliciting stories from members of ONS and other oncology-affiliated organizations. We disseminated the request for stories to our patients, colleagues, and other personal and professional contacts. Thanks to the typing skills of Sue Hines, Barb Fersch, and Peggy Smith, we were able to keep up with analysis of the stories for selection. We read each story we received carefully and gave it a numerical rating based on a score sheet we developed. We compared our scores with those of the Oncology Nursing Press Silver Linings team, and we were pleased that we generally agreed upon which stories would best send the message of Silver Linings. When we were not in complete agreement on the stories, we requested input from our husbands, Joe Gullo and Steve Glass, and our friends, Loretta Ward, Pid Dickey, and other nursing colleagues. They provided us with yet another perspective as representatives of the general public, survivors of cancer, or nursing colleagues. Selecting a limited number of stories for final publication was difficult because each story brought out a unique and new dimension of the cancer experience.

We began the first part of the editing process fortified by the Silver Linings team from the Oncology Nursing Press, which included Vikki Newton, managing editor; Lisa George, Jen Krause, and Sharon Dougherty, copy editors; and Tracey Vaccarello, editorial assistant. They helped us to bring out the "silver" in each story, which was our continuing goal. We accomplished this according to a mutually agreed upon time frame established with the guidance of

Anne Snively, production manager. The layout process was another team effort as we collaborated with Jim Morton, creative services associate, Maria Gamiere, illustrator, and the entire team. We wish to give special acknowledgment to Jan Kinzler and Vikki Newton, who were always offering encouragement and insight along the way.

The talented artist Maria Gamiere provided art work that was a creative gift to the project. She skillfully weaved her art around the selected stories. We appreciate her talent, patience, and grace as she combined our suggestions into visual illustrations. She donated countless hours to complete the final art, which provided rich illustrations for this unique book of hope. Maria's husband, Mick, and her mother, Caterina, are both cancer survivors, which increased Maria's astute sensitivity to the stories she was illustrating.

Throughout the entire process, our families provided us with emotional support and time to persevere through the many hours required to complete the book. We shared many working weekends, which began at predawn and ended at midnight. The inspiration from the stories buoyed our tired bodies and minds as we saw the book taking form. Long telephone calls helped us to blend our skills and ideas in the manuscript preparation. Each step of the journey we became more excited as we realized the promise of hope and meaning the book would bring to those with cancer, their loved ones, and the many dedicated professionals caring for and about them.

Because of the complexity of this project, we may have inadvertently left out the names of some of the people who also helped us. If so, we apologize, but please know that we appreciated your insight, your caring, your support, and your assistance.

We wish to acknowledge the 900+ cancer survivors, family members, friends, nurses, and others who contributed their stories. They cared enough to share their time and innermost feelings in their stories. They honestly communicated all facets of emotions one deals with when diagnosed with cancer. With rare exception, they all expressed the desire to help others going through the cancer experience. Without them, this book would not have been possible. They are true heros and heroines of *Silver Linings: The Other Side of Cancer.*

Shirley M. Gullo
Elaine Glass

Introduction

Silver Linings: The Other Side of Cancer is a unique book that shares the insights and comforting words of people who have experienced cancer. As oncology nurses, we've seen how the dark cloud of cancer often holds a silver lining—lessons learned through the cancer experience make life easier, richer, happier, and more meaningful. The stories describe the lessons that helped survivors through their darkest moments to find new perspectives on life that led to peace, serenity, and even joy. Their messages provide insight on ways to cope effectively and transcend the cloud of cancer.

The stories are written by people from all walks of life, demonstrating that cancer shows no respect for age, gender, social class, or race. *Silver Linings* stories are grouped into seven chapters based on the main theme of the story. The editors have tried to keep the authors' narratives intact as much as possible to maintain the full intent of their messages; however, they have edited stories to enhance clarity and to meet space requirements. Stories are adorned with illustrations or quotes to highlight or enhance the focus of the story.

The first chapter, "Caught in the Storm," identifies the initial battle with cancer and the patterns of healing that follow. One survivor writes, "After I was diagnosed with breast cancer, there were so many things that I saw differently; yet, nothing about them had actually changed! I had changed. Although I didn't look different, I was profoundly different. I mean, how could I not be? A person cannot face a potentially fatal disease and not be somehow changed." Another writes, "My cancer reinforced some of my deepest values—or it was a powerful confirmation of what really matters in life. I say embrace Life and not Death." They are stories of finding new strengths and continuing life with a new enthusiasm.

The second chapter, "Love: The Best Umbrella," deals with enhanced romantic love or love of friends and others. One writer describes how devastated she felt following a mastectomy, yet how very loved she felt after hearing her husband's healing words: "There is nothing that could make me stop loving you. You are the love of my life!" Others describe the love they felt from others who reached out to them in time of need.

One author writes, "My most glowing silver lining is the renewed closeness, depth, and mutual appreciation that has developed between me and those dearest to me." She adds, "Whatever happens in the future, I will go forward knowing that I am loved, I have touched and been touched by many lives and loves."

The chapter "Family Ties Reach Beyond Gray Skies" describes the new strengths that can develop within families as a result of experiencing the many life changes from cancer. One writer states, "Cancer teaches a family how to react to the valleys in life"; others describe how a family may be fortified by the cancer experience. Another story reveals how priorities may change: "Times with family members are irreplaceable and the stuff my happiness is made of. Now I try to make these opportunities rather than wait for them to happen."

As those with cancer reach out to others who have gone through similar experiences, they often find a revitalized strength through newly formed friendships with fellow travelers on the road of cancer or others who have reached out to offer help. The fourth chapter, "Personal Connections: A Guiding Light Through the Cancer Experience," focuses on these connections. As one writer expresses, "I think sometimes it is harder to be the one who loves the patient than to be the patient. The role of standing by is a difficult one. I realize what a gift it was to others when I permitted them to assist me. Preparing a meal, washing clothes, car pooling, sending a card—all of these tangible signs of love and intention connected us together." Emerging groups are using the Internet to reach out to others with cancer through new technologies. Another author encouraged others to "just reach out, turn on your computer, and open up a whole new world!"

Chapter 5, "Style and Wit: A Compass Toward Healing," is filled with humorous stories and quotes from those who have discovered wit to be one of their greatest assets. "Humor can hasten the healing"; "When anger and pain mount, one gentle nudge from humor restores balance. In a very profound way, humor makes life worth living." These words come to life in stories such as the tale about the man who was embarrassed about having to undress in front of the female radiation technicians during his treatments. His wife and friends came to the rescue, and each of his radiation treatments triggered laughs by the staff and other patients. Please read about how he dealt with his embarrassment in a humorous way to help him gain control of the situation.

Chapter 6, "Cherish the Rainbows," provides valuable lessons for everyone as it points to the importance of appreciating each moment of our lives. One contributor states, "Early in life, my mother taught me about the quest for silver linings: It is both a skill and a mental attitude. Cancer's silver lining is that it fuels our hunt for other silver linings more intensely than ever." A 12-year survivor of breast cancer explains, "Illness is a great teacher. I have learned to be kinder to myself." Another author shares these thoughts: "My days are no longer ordinary. They are bright and full of new and exciting things. Cancer takes ordinary people and teaches them to be extraordinary. I am now a cheerleading squad of one that cheers and encourages other survivors to be all they can be."

The final chapter illustrates what is, for many, the heart of the cancer experience. Throughout many of the stories in "Spiritual Discoveries: The True Silver Lining," the substance of faith comforted and sustained many patients and families when everything else seemed bleak and hopeless. One young survivor writes, "In the big picture, we are but a heartbeat on a planet of billions. Don't tolerate small complaints such as the sun not coming out. Sometimes it is just hidden. Sometimes the love of God is hidden, too." A bone marrow transplant survivor described her feelings: "I was supported on a cushion of prayers offered by family, friends, and people I did not even know. I have learned to more fully and deeply appreciate the meaning and possibilities of my life."

Silver Linings is a beautiful book of radiance; it is richly illustrated in colorful and creative art woven from the illustrator's and the authors' lives. These are encouraging stories of triumph, miracles, families rebuilding their lives, humor, and people finding strength and faith they never knew they had. There are few simple answers in life. These touching, moving stories reveal the steps along cancer's stormy pathway—steps that can lead others to look for and find the glints of light and hope that are the silver linings of life in the dark clouds of cancer.

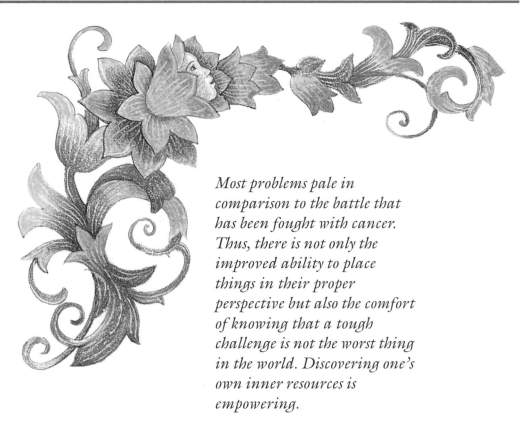

Most problems pale in comparison to the battle that has been fought with cancer. Thus, there is not only the improved ability to place things in their proper perspective but also the comfort of knowing that a tough challenge is not the worst thing in the world. Discovering one's own inner resources is empowering.

Jane Llewellyn, DNSc, RN
*Nurse administrator and
breast cancer survivor
Illinois*

Chapter 1

Caught in the Storm

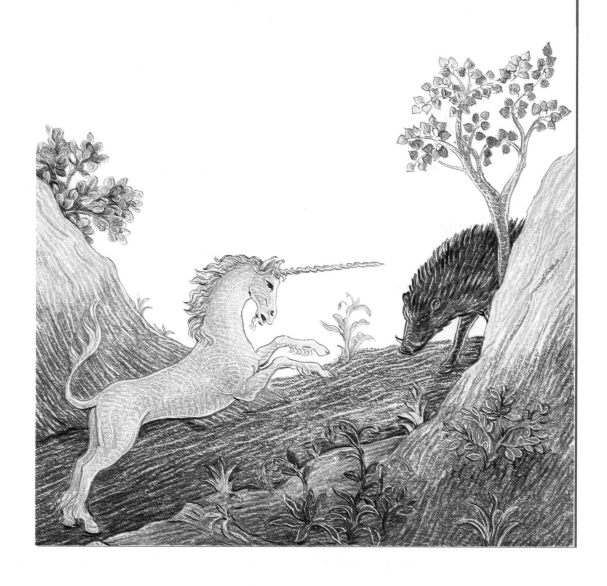

The Wrong Side of Cancer

In writing these words, I discovered that the most important things in life are love and understanding.

When I first heard about the book project *Silver Linings: The Other Side of Cancer,* I realized that I was on the wrong side. What can be said of cancer except that it can kill you? Look at my lovely wife. Because of my cancer, she has endured the worst this illness can dish out.

As I sat down to write this, I reflected. I found out that a lot can be said about what we have gone through—good and bad, but mostly good. Folks have heard all the negatives. They are typical of a catastrophic illness such as cancer. I wonder, though, if you've heard how much closer you become with your loved ones as a result of this disease? How many times have you shared your expressions of love—to your wife and to your God? Cancer can be deadly, but it forces you to make peace with God. It gives you time to rekindle old and lost friendships. You can make restitution and settle some old debts.

Yes, I made it to the other side of the lining. I followed the rainbow to a pot—not filled with gold but with love, understanding, and support. I know now how much everyone loves me. I thought that writing about the silver linings was going to be depressing, but it's not. In writing these words, I discovered that the most important things in life are love and understanding.

I'm here to tell you today, don't quit! Don't get discouraged! Look for these things of love I have spoken of today. How ironic this is—I didn't really see these things until I sat down to write.

God bless you all.

Tom T.Y. Yessler
Ohio

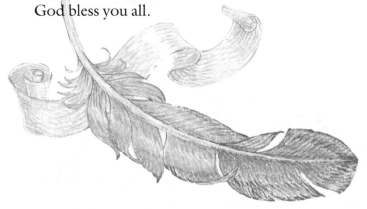

Attitude Is More Important Than Facts

Having cancer hasn't been all bad. It has certainly strengthened my soul.

In March of 1995, I lost my job with the newspaper. One week later, I found a lump in my breast. The doctor immediately diagnosed it as malignant. My husband of 30 years walked out the door. "You know I don't like to be around sick people," said my semisenile 85-year-old mother.

I remember how frightened and alone I felt as I sat in my surgeon's office listening to my pathology report. Emotionally and physically, I stood touching the rocks at the bottom. The next week, I met with my wonderful oncologist in Colorado Springs. I will never forget his kindness and encouragement. He gave me hope with the promise of a bone marrow transplant. Suddenly, I knew I would survive.

"God, you may have to carry me occasionally, but, with your help, I can beat this," I said aloud in my car while driving home.

Next, I began reading books written by cancer survivors. I started drinking eight glasses of water daily. I counted fat calories and made sure I ate at least five fresh fruits and five fresh vegetable servings each day. I began an exercise program. I meditated daily. In short, I did everything I could to help myself.

Having cancer hasn't been all bad. It has certainly strengthened my soul. Today, I work as a "Reach to Recovery" volunteer. Through this, I have met many totally dedicated people.

In Dr. Karl Menninger's words, "Attitude is more important than facts."

Eleanor McKee
Breast cancer survivor
Hawaii

Because of You, I Took the Helicopter

I'm not afraid. God will save me.

As an oncology staff nurse at a hospital, I had patients who were diagnosed with colon cancer. One beautiful, religious lady was having a hard time with the decision of facing life with a colostomy. She actually was in the process of giving up and deciding against any surgery. Underneath her reluctance was the fear that her husband would not love her anymore. I gave her a lot of emotional support and shared a funny story that I had read in *Reader's Digest*. I had to tell the story quickly because I was being paged. It went something like this:

It rained for days. The rivers were beginning to overflow their banks. The authorities issued an official flood warning. Announcements were made on radio and TV about evacuation routes and rescue efforts. As the sheriff drove by one man's house, he yelled for the man to get out while there was still time. The man refused, stating that God would take care of him. A few hours later, two guys went by the man's house in a rowboat and noticed that he was sitting in the second-story window. They offered him a ride in their boat. The man again professed his faith that God would take care of him. By the next morning, the man was atop his roof, clutching his chimney. A helicopter pilot called down from overhead and told him to grab hold of the rope and they would pull him aboard. The man replied, "I'm not afraid, God will save me."

Later on that day, the man's body was found floating down the river. Upon facing God in Heaven, the man asked God why He had let him drown. God replied, "I sent a car, a boat, and a helicopter. What more did you want?"

Several weeks later, this woman returned to the unit to tell me that, after thinking about the story I had told her, she had decided to have the surgery. The procedure was successful, and she recuperated well. She gave me a book titled *Don't Just Stand There, Pray Something*.

Inside the book was a note that read, "Because of you, I took the helicopter. Thanks for suggesting that it would be a good flight."

Since then, I occasionally see this woman in my local drugstore. She always says, "Thank you for the helicopter." I had no idea the humorous story would have such an impact.

Delores Belvin, RN, OCN®
Oncology nurse
Florida

As I waited in radiology, I encountered a man with one leg amputated. He walked down the hall on crutches. I decided this encounter was God's helping hand extended to me, as if to say "Get a grip and hang on."

Mary Barry, RN
Breast cancer survivor, wife, mother of four, and nurse
Ohio

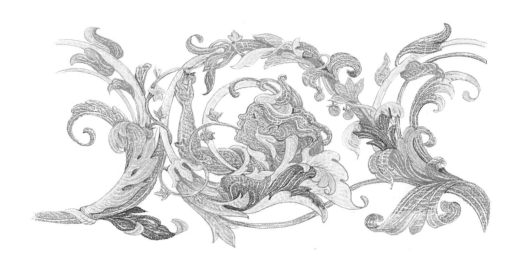

Impossibilities

Hope is indeed manifested in the courage to keep trying despite overwhelming odds.

In the late 1980s, when my clinical nurse specialist position became more outpatient- and community-focused, my office moved to the radiation oncology department. Similar to most outpatient radiation therapy centers, ours saw a high volume of patients and families come and go each day. It was a busy and, at times, quite hectic department. Numerous administrative and support staff members were needed to care for the more than 100 patients treated daily.

One afternoon, I was on the phone in my office adjacent to the waiting room when I heard an unusually high volume of chatter and raised voices out by the reception desk. I ignored it at first, but then the intensity of the sounds escalated, almost to a chant of mini squeals. Deciding to investigate, I walked into the waiting area to find every female in the department clustered around a most unusual sight— a three-seat stroller carrying the most adorable set of infant triplet boys I had ever seen. In fact, I had never seen a set of triplets before! Incredibly, at the helm of this unique baby carriage was a patient we had treated for Hodgkin's disease years before. She had received an aggressive course of chemotherapy *plus* total body irradiation. At the time of her initial diagnosis and subsequent treatment, she was told that these combined therapies without doubt cause infertility. Here she was. Not only did she have nine-month-old triplets following her cancer treatment, but she conceived them without the help of any fertility drugs! My jaw immediately dropped to my knees!

After this amazing scene, I asked a gynecologist colleague about the chances of this occurring. He stated that in a "normal" population, it was a one-in-a-million chance for this type of pregnancy to occur. He then said that he could not even begin to postulate what the likelihood was for a cancer survivor who had undergone such intensive treatment as our patient had received.

Although this is a somewhat extreme example, it is indicative of experiences many of us in the cancer field have had over time. In more than 25 years as an oncology nurse, I have witnessed so many exceptions to the rule. I now know why most physicians continue to offer hope to patients, even in the most dire of circumstances. There are always those patients who fool us. Even with questionable prognoses, people can respond to treatment with amazing success and live beyond our greatest expectations. This incident, and others, just prove to me that our conventional clinical wisdom only holds true for some. Hope should be a mainstay of all cancer-related discussions, for we professionals don't know all the answers, nor should we profess to. Hope is indeed manifested in the courage to keep trying despite overwhelming odds.

Deborah McCaffrey Boyle, RN, MSN, OCN®
Cancer nurse specialist
Virginia

Fear, anger, vulnerability, and hopelessness are words often associated with cancer. Other feelings, however, also are expressed, such as hope, peacefulness, an enriched life, and growth.

Mary Earle Young
Wisconsin

Passing the Flame of Life

She was rejuvenated through prayer, family,
and her strong will to live.

Susie and I were married on October 6, 1984. Three years later, we were blessed with our son, Ryan, born February 5, 1987, and two years later, our daughter, Natalie, was born on May 16, 1989. Both were healthy, and that's what mattered! Our priorities were spending time together, camping, motorcycling, and engaging in other family-oriented activities when I wasn't working at Aber's Truck Center as a mechanic.

We were living the All-American Dream until April 1994, when our lives suddenly changed. Susie thought she just had the flu and figured it would run its course. After a month of feeling ill, she decided to seek medical treatment. She was immediately sent to the hospital and was admitted with a diagnosis of acute leukemia. Since this is one of the fastest-acting cancers, time was of the essence. Leukemia cells take over the blood in your body. They prohibit the blood cells and platelets from carrying out their functions. This leaves you open to infection because you can't fight off even everyday germs. You also have a greater chance of bleeding when your platelets are low.

Late that first night in the hospital, nurses struggled to find veins for blood transfusions to stabilize Susie. She received eight units of blood and six units of platelets. Her body was drained from leukemia. Susie brushed the door of death late that night. My eyes were open wide, my mouth dragging the floor. Susie showed us her courage and will to live. God showed us that He was there and wasn't ready for her yet. She made it through the night. The doctor on call said Susie needed to be at a larger hospital, so she was transferred to Cleveland Clinic the next day.

The doctors and nursing staff tried to put us at ease, schooling us through each procedure. They ran many tests over the next two days. An IV line for chemotherapy was placed in her chest. The drugs were too strong to be administered in the veins of her arms, and the doctors needed more than one place to hook up to. Susie then underwent a bone marrow biopsy, a procedure done by drawing blood and marrow from the hip bone. The bone marrow is where all blood is produced in the body. The procedure helps identify the extent of leukemia. Since 90% of Susie's bone marrow was filled with leukemia, her chemotherapy started only five days after the diagnosis. It ran for seven days and caused very few side effects. She felt quite good, had only a few fevers, and had a skin rash.

Six days later, the second bone marrow biopsy revealed that the chemotherapy had no effect on the leukemia. A second round of treatment was necessary. Another seven days! This time, our children stayed with my parents and two sisters. During this second round of chemotherapy, the side effects started setting in—nausea, rashes from the medications, fevers, and hair loss. Support and prayer seemed to be the only things that kept us going.

The third bone marrow biopsy revealed no good and no bad cells. Time would be the answer. Susie struggled through the side effects. Her rash looked like she had been burned with fire; her arms and legs were swollen to the size of footballs.

After waiting 35 days, a fourth bone marrow biopsy revealed that all the new blood cells were again leukemic. A third round of chemotherapy would be necessary. It was her only hope now! This chemotherapy would be four times her body weight or the highest amount she could take. Throughout this time, Susie received support from cards, prayers, faith, and family. Her strength, a vital part of fighting the battle, was beginning to fade. The separation from her family made the devastation settle deeper each day. The high-dose chemotherapy was supposed to run six days. After the fourth day, her body said no more. Susie stood to be weighed and collapsed. She lost all her motor functions. She couldn't walk or talk. The doctor said they would stop the chemotherapy and wait to see if the side effects would go away. Time would tell.

The fifth bone marrow biopsy was taken six days after they stopped the treatment. It revealed no good or bad cells—"Empty," they said. Twenty-eight days went by before any cells could be detected, but not enough cells were present to tell for sure whether they were good or bad cells. While fighting the side effects, Susie brushed the door of death two more times during these 28 days. The drugs had to fight off all the germs because her body couldn't. She was dangling by a string. By this time, because her appetite was very low, she had lost 26 pounds and had to be fed through her IV catheter. Struggling through each day, Susie began to regain some of her motor functions. She was rejuvenated through prayer, family, and her strong will to live.

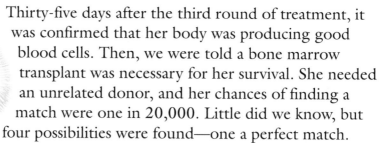

Thirty-five days after the third round of treatment, it was confirmed that her body was producing good blood cells. Then, we were told a bone marrow transplant was necessary for her survival. She needed an unrelated donor, and her chances of finding a match were one in 20,000. Little did we know, but four possibilities were found—one a perfect match.

After three-and-one-half months in the hospital, Susie was able to come home on August 7, 1994, to recover from her ordeal.

After seven weeks at home, her strength, courage, and some motor function began returning. On October 3, 1994, she returned to the hospital for a bone marrow transplant. She had to go through an extensive seven-day chemotherapy regimen to prepare her body for it. Susie received her bone marrow transplant October 13, 1994. It was little more than a sandwich bag full and took only minutes to run through her main line.

The results of her first bone marrow biopsy reflected good cell growth from the new bone marrow. It was a really great match! Susie was released on October 28—only 25 days after her transplant. She is truly a miracle, all thanks to prayer, family, and God Himself.

One-and-a-half years after Susie's bone marrow transplant, she was nominated by the Cleveland Clinic staff to carry the Olympic Torch in the cross-country relay. Thanks to The National Bone Marrow Registry, Coca-Cola, and the hospital, the arrangements were made. Susie was so excited to have this great honor. And, she passed the torch in St. Paul, MN, to her bone marrow donor Barb LeCleir, from Eau Claire, WI.

Thomas L. Wells
Husband of Susie Wells, bone marrow transplant survivor
Ohio

Don't give up,
Dig deeper down—and in.
Everyone's in your corner,
Cheering you on across the line to
WIN!

Anthony Taylor
Son of mother with breast cancer
Texas

The View From Remission

Look up high and what do you see?
Dark clouds of cancer hanging over me.
Recurrence and death, two clouds of doom'
Grief and fear add to the gloom.

Yet, look all around me: It's clear and bright!
Because lining each cloud is a silvery light,
A glow so strong it reveals the way
peace and joy can infuse life every day.

I accept the uncertainty and lack of control,
But I still miss the innocence my illness stole.
I hate cancer scares, canceling plans,
and feeling anxious while awaiting scans.
But . . . I love

The Silver Linings

A valuable education in illness and healing granted few physicians.
A new career in writing, a different but equal passion and a way to reach
more people than I ever could in my medical office.
A few unexpected years at home with my children, during which I've
embraced the parenting I could do each day, maybe doing a better job
than I would have done with all the time in the world.
Many old relationships made richer for having shared trying times,
incredible new friendships that would never have been born otherwise,
and an ever-deepening spiritual faith.

The knowledge of what might have been lost (and might yet be)
makes me feel today, every day, in a wonderfully intense way. Little
problems remain trivial. The ordinary has become marvelous. I seek out
and cherish joyful moments. Even unpleasant times are less painful, for
they are proof that I am still here.

Wendy S. Harpham, MD
Author of After Cancer, Diagnosis Cancer,
When a Parent Has Cancer, and Becky and the Worry Cup
Texas

The Deal With God

I was told that I will have to take medicine the rest of my life. I was afraid to ask, "How many days are you writing the prescription for?"

At the age of 22, I had a partial thyroidectomy. A cancerous tumor the size of a walnut was surgically removed from my thyroid. I was told that I needed to have follow-up scans for five years and would have to take medicine the rest of my life. I was afraid to ask, "How many days are you writing the prescription for?"

I wasn't quite sure what to make of the situation. I felt I had no one to talk to about my life. My father had died of a heart attack two years before my surgery, and my mother was in a deep state of depression. I felt very alone and frightened and didn't know where to turn. So, I was left with one resource my parents had given to me—I talked to God. I made a deal with Him that if He would let me live until I was 35, get married, have children, and experience life as a wife and mother, I would then turn my life over to Him.

So, for the next few years, I tried to make the most of my life and realize some of my dreams. These dreams included getting married, having two children, graduating from college, living in Taiwan, and traveling to Hong Kong, Australia, New Zealand, Fiji, and Europe. My life was very rich and full of wonderful people.

At the age of 35, I was wondering if I would get the "call" from God, but instead I was given a project. My mother was ill and needed nursing home care. As I muddled through the healthcare system with her, I decided to make a career change from finance to social work. It sounds strange, and people often tell me that having an MBA and an MSW is quite an unusual combination. However, I was fortunate enough to put these two credentials to work. In 1991, I received a social work fellowship from the American Cancer Society at Children's National Medical Center in Washington, DC, to work with families whose children have cancer.

While I was at Children's, my brother's four-year-old son was diagnosed with leukemia. When my brother called, I was at a loss for words. We both cried. That was five years ago. My nephew is nine years old now and is doing very well. Recently, I turned 47! Our family has so much to be thankful for.

My career now is in social work. I work at a cancer center facilitating support groups for adult patients with cancer and their families. I also coordinate a program for children whose parents are in cancer treatment or whose parents have died of cancer. Recently, I started a support group for siblings of children with cancer. Cancer is now part of my life in another way—helping children deal with the emotional roller coaster when a loved one has been diagnosed with cancer.

Thanks to my husband, children, family, and friends, I have a very rewarding life. I hope you, too, find your silver lining.

Karen Kostreba
Cancer survivor
Virginia

The dictionary describes a survivor as someone who remains alive after, or in spite of, a mortally dangerous occurrence or situation. So, whether you survive the ride home after work on a busy freeway or are one of only a few who walked out of a bombed-out building in Oklahoma City, you are a survivor. Keeping this thought in mind, we are all survivors. We must all celebrate and appreciate the time that is given to us. I like to think that our diagnosis of cancer gives us an edge over everyone else. We are acutely aware of and appreciate the time we have and strive to make others see how precious life can be.

Carole McGlochin
Four-year survivor of ovarian cancer
Colorado

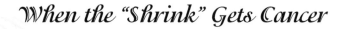

When the "Shrink" Gets Cancer

As a nurse and psychotherapist working with people with cancer for over 25 years, I had never considered myself to be immune from developing cancer and had often wondered how I would cope if it suddenly became "my turn." Well, I recently found out, in the midst of preparations to lecture in Shanghai and Hong Kong on topics such as "Communication and Breaking Bad News." We were traveling abroad as a family of four—my husband, Bruce, 26-year-old son, Wolfgang, and 17-year-old daughter, Alexa. Bruce, Alexa, and I have traveled frequently as I lectured throughout the world, but we hadn't traveled as a family of four before.

Wolfgang had left home at age 14, one month into ninth grade, and had become a street kid. Last June, after dropping out of school 12 years earlier, he graduated with distinction from college, earning a degree in drama and education. We were traveling to do workshops together on anger, anticipatory loss and grief, and grief and bereavement. Needless to say, the trip was very special.

Three weeks before the trip, I had an ultrasound to diagnose the source of some minor abdominal pain that I thought was an ulcer. It turned out to be lymphoma. I was surprised but explained to the doctors that they would have to get on with things quickly as I needed to travel. The team really worked together to help me to achieve my goals. Surgery, a bone marrow biopsy, and chemotherapy were quickly coordinated. I received chemotherapy on Monday, and we left for Shanghai on Thursday—loaded with drugs to keep me symptom-free.

The trip was great. The morning after we arrived, I had a breakfast of congee (Chinese porridge) with pickled vegetables, but I passed on the century-old eggs. We ate more wonderful 10-course Chinese meals than I could count and were treated royally. The lectures and workshops were a great success—although Wolfgang said that watching his mother lecture while her hair gradually fell out was a bit unnerving. However, my hair cooperated a little and stayed around for a few extra days as I finished my lecture tour and gave a local lecture to palliative care physicians.

I finished treatment five and have begun classes in relaxation and meditation—yoga and qi gong. I am continuing my clinical work and feel almost normal. I have spoken with most of my clients on a "need-to-know basis." I've offered them the option of seeing someone else if my diagnosis upset them. Without exception, they have wished me well, asked some questions about my health, and proceeded to deal with the issues that brought them to me in the first place. A few have even offered the suggestion that it will make me an even better therapist, not—they hasten to add—that I had been less than a perfect therapist before.

Mary L.S. Vachon, RN, PhD
Consultant in psychosocial oncology and palliative care
Ontario, Canada

Keep a level head. Don't yield to the emotionality of the cancer experience. Resist having magical expectations of "miracle" drugs. Instead, ask for honest information about side effects of proposed treatments so you can weigh them against the proposed benefits. Ironically, it seems that facing every aspect of cancer head-on, with realistic expectations, neutralizes fear and vulnerability. This head-on approach leads, ultimately, to control and peace of mind.

Mary Earle Young
Wisconsin

A Few Words on Cancer

DAY 1

CANCER   ME   NO   MISTAKE

WEEK 1

SCARED   ALONE   ANXIOUS

WEEK 2

STUDY   LEARN   READ   ASK

SUPPORT   ENCOURAGEMENT   GOD   HELP   VITALITY

DREAM   LIFE   GRANDCHILDREN   TRAVEL

NORMAL

MONTH 1

NURSE   SURGEON   PROCEDURE   RESECTION

CATHETER

ENDURE   HOPE   OPTIMISM   FAITH

GOD

YEAR 1

CHEMOTHERAPY   PRAYER   VISUALIZE   ACTUALIZE

FAVORABLE   CONSOLIDATION   6,400 RADS

FINISHED

WAIT   WATCH   SEE   HOPE   PRAY

YEAR 2

VOLUNTEER   HELP   SUPPORT

AMERICAN CANCER SOCIETY   BIOPSIES

RECURRENCE IMMUNOTHERAPY SUFFERING ENDURE

HAPPIER   FRIENDLIER   CHEERFUL

LOVE   BUTTERFLIES   NEVER GIVE UP

TODAY   THANK GOD

TOMORROW   MAYBE

NO MATTER

TODAY   ENJOY   TODAY

PLEASE GOD   SILVER LININGS

THANKS GOD

Frederick A. Hesketh
New proud grandfather reacting to invasive bladder cancer; author of In Control: A Cancer Victim Describes His Struggle to Gain Control of the Mind and the Body
Connecticut

"C" stands for cancer, *but it is only one letter on life.*

Anthony Taylor
Son of mother with breast cancer
Texas

I have been in remission for six years. There are still times when I am angry and scared. Every year that passes takes a little bit more anger and fear away with it. I move closer to a mental and emotional remission—one day at a time. My life is good. I am a cancer survivor.

Katie Gill
Six-year survivor of Hodgkin's disease
Ohio

The Poem and the President

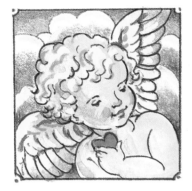

Pray and be strong is all I can do. I can be scared, and so can you.

Presumably, when Kelly Shaw wrote the poem to her mother about her fears about cancer and her mother's possible death, she never thought anyone else would read it, let alone the President of the United States.

"I can really only write (poems) when I'm feeling really sad," said Shaw, 16, a high school sophomore. "It's my emotion . . . I have to really be feeling it."

Goodbye
Wondering when we will have to say goodbye,
All I can do is cry.
Waking up in the middle of the night,
and trying to fight . . . ,
all of the tears, like an uncontrollable kite.
I have never had to depart
from someone so close to my heart.
When you become an angel,
there is no coming back,
yet the memories of you will never lack . . .

For nearly half of Kelly's life, she has been feeling the conflicting emotions of watching her mother, Marcie Hahn, battle cancer. Marcie first was diagnosed with breast cancer at the age of 33. She was in remission for four years before doctors discovered the cancer in her bones. Again, she refused to concede and battled the disease a second time, gaining another four years of remission.

Just last month, Marcie came out of remission again when, during a routine checkup, doctors found the cancer had metastasized to a bone in her leg and soft tissue in her back. "Here I am, battling it again," said the unflappable Marcie. Marcie resigned herself to more chemotherapy, but her daughter took on the disease in a different way, through her poetry.

"I'm so proud of the fact that she's able to put her feelings onto paper.

It's so therapeutic," said Marcie, who, as it turns out, copes with her own feelings through her job at the Cancer Wellness Center.

The morning after Kelly wrote the poem and gave it to her mother, they learned of the death of President Bill Clinton's mother, Virginia Kelley, after a long battle with breast cancer.

"That poem touched me so much," said Marcie. "I had to share it with (the Clintons)." She drafted a letter to the Clintons and enclosed a copy of Kelly's poem.

Several weeks later, the president visited Wright Community College in Chicago to speak on healthcare reform. Kelly and her mom attended. After the speech, Secret Service men approached them and ushered them to a back room to meet the president. Marcie said she was speechless.

Kelly had no such awe—she chatted easily with the president. "He thanked me for the poem and said he was really touched," said Kelly. "He was really nice to talk to. I wasn't uncomfortable at all." In fact, she was so relaxed she remembered to ask him for an autograph. On the poem, of course.

The woman who raised me to the girl I am today,
is the bravest woman, if I may say
You are fighting for you, and you are fighting for me.
I'll make you the proudest mom, just wait and see . . .

If the angels take you now, you can send me messages.
How?
By ringing me bells and kissing my cells,
cancer free . . .

I hope I never inherit this unfair disease,
but if I do, I will accept it with ease.
Pray and be strong, is all I can do.
I can be scared, and so can you.
We will leave it up to God,
He will fight for you too.

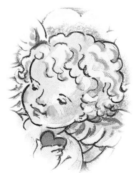

From "Poem Puts Teen, Clinton on Common Ground,"
by Eileen O. Daday. Reprinted from the March 14, 1994 issue
by permission of the Daily Herald, *Arlington Heights, IL*

Lucky 13

The nurses told me that my positive attitude helped me get well.

I was diagnosed with lymphoma in October of 1964. I was 35 years old. In 1964, very little was known about lymphoma. The little bit of news that I did receive from the doctor in Middletown, OH, was not good. My family and I were very concerned. I had a wife and four young sons to take care of. I couldn't die and leave them to fend for themselves.

I was sent to The Ohio State University Hospitals in Columbus for more tests and a medical plan recommending what to do. They sent me back home to receive 10 radiation treatments at Middletown Hospital. This was the only treatment known at the time. We hoped and prayed that it would work. The tumors went away and I was healthy again. I returned to my work as an electrician.

Approximately 13 years later in 1976, during a routine checkup, another tumor was found. This time, the doctor had good news. Several treatments for my lymphoma were now available. After a staging laparotomy, I received a year of experimental chemotherapy and immune therapy. I lost all my hair and was quite weak at times. However, I wasn't going to let this lymphoma get me. I beat it once. I was going to beat it again.

Two things helped me in my fight against the lymphoma. One, I never made a career out of being a patient. I wouldn't let myself slip into the "poor me" syndrome. I often made myself go to work, even when I was quite weak. I hardly ever missed a day.

The second thing that helped me through was my determination to act "normal." For me, this was having fun and making people laugh. To prove to myself and others that I was a normal, fun guy, I'd fly my 182 Cessna airplane the 90 miles from Middletown to Columbus to get my chemotherapy treatments. Sometimes, one of my neighbors would fly up with me if her appointment fell on the same day.

I was especially good at making people laugh. I love to tell jokes. I found out that doctors and nurses appreciated a good chuckle in the middle of a hectic work day. I discovered, too, that if you can keep yourself and others laughing and in a good mood, the cancer isn't so scary. Cancer can't get to you as easily when you're up. My nurses confirmed this when they told me that my positive attitude helped me get well. After a year of chemotherapy, the tumors went away for a second time and I was healthy again.

Then, almost another 13 years later in 1990, I discovered a tumor on the back of my neck. Even better news this time. After the tumor was removed by the surgeon, no further treatment was needed. All the rest of my tests showed that there was no cancer anywhere else in my body. My own immune system was keeping the lymphoma under control.

Since then, I have been going every six months for checkups. I know there are now a lot of good treatments for lymphoma if mine decides to come back on me again in 2003—when I'm 72. I'm living proof that it is possible to survive for years with cancer. I'm now on year #33 and still going strong.

I thank God for answering all the prayers of my family and friends and for my health. I also appreciate all the dedicated doctors and nurses at The James Cancer Hospital and Research Institute for their caring and concerning ways—and for laughing at my crazy jokes.

Gail A. Sickle
Husband and father with lymphoma
Florida

When you look at all of it together, it's a mountain. When you just take each step as it comes, it's an attainable summit.

Brandon Creger
Osteosarcoma survivor
Michigan

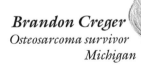

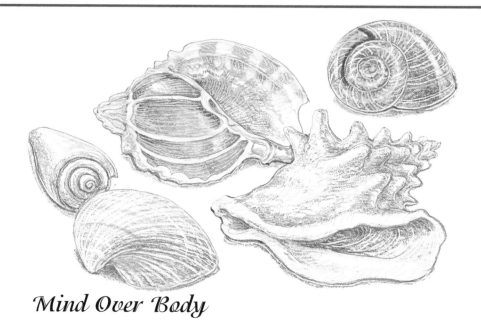

Mind Over Body

The power of the mind over the body is truly incredible.

After my sister's death from leukemia, my mother feared all her aches and pains were from cancers traveling through her body. Thirteen years of panic came true with her diagnosis of breast cancer. She feared she lacked the inner strength to fight the cancer, but she surprised herself by completing six months of treatment with a positive attitude. The cancer was gone from her body.

Over the next two years, my mother feared recurrence of her disease. Two years after her initial diagnosis, back and abdominal pain led to the diagnosis of metastatic breast cancer to the pancreas, adrenal gland, and small intestine. My mother now had "traveling cancer." During a heart-to-heart talk, I asked her if she believed her persistent image of "traveling cancer" contributed to her diagnosis. When she answered "I don't know . . . maybe," I asked if she would be willing to practice guided imagery in conjunction with her chemotherapy and bone marrow transplant. Initially reluctant to try anything requiring concentration, she finally agreed.

Without formal training, I began with some basic techniques I acquired in school. I asked her to close her eyes, think of her favorite place, put herself there, and listen to the sounds. She told me she could see and feel herself at her favorite beach on Cape Cod. With my guidance, she imagined the waves from the ocean sweeping over her abdomen and taking the tumors out to sea. Each passing wave smoothed out her "bumpy" tumors, and the sea gulls helped by pecking away at the remains.

Now that we found my mother's source of inner strength, we bought tapes of ocean sounds from various musical artists. These tapes helped guide her images when alone and during chemotherapy.

Initially, Mom feared a rapid and painful death. Later, she felt an inner strength to conquer her cancer and beat the odds. "I won't be another statistic!" she said.

Later, my mother developed intestinal complications and required two major surgeries and six weeks of hospitalization. Unable to focus on her once therapeutic guided imagery, she began losing her inner strength. "I don't want to die, but I can't do this anymore," she said. "If this is living, I would rather die." After much encouragement, I reintroduced imagery for relaxation and mind-over-body control. While everything else felt out of her control, guided imagery helped her realize what she could do for herself. She focused her images on sending in extra sea gulls to peck away at the obstruction so she could continue her treatment.

A CAT scan, taken before her second surgery, remarkably revealed no detectable masses on any organ. We believe guided imagery has strongly contributed to shrinking the tumors after only two doses of chemotherapy. Mom still has a bumpy road of treatment ahead, and guided imagery will continue to help her to realize her life dreams.

My mother found the inner strength to conquer her fears that she once thought were impossible to fight. She continues impressing our whole family, her doctors, and most importantly, herself. The power of the mind over the body is truly incredible!

Lisa St. Amand
Bone marrow transplant nurse
Massachusetts

Cancer has opened many new doors for me. I don't know where my journey may lead me, but I plan on making the most I can on this path.

Elaine Metzung
Mother of three young children and breast cancer survivor
Ohio

Bone Marrow Transplant Pioneer

Without a doubt, Mushtaque Jivani, 47, is a bone marrow transplantation (BMT) pioneer in every sense of the word. When he was diagnosed with acute myeloid leukemia in October 1976 at age 27, the prognosis for the disease was grim. Upon delivering the diagnosis, Mushtaque's physician told him he was "going to die today, tomorrow, or in a week" and suggested that Mushtaque get his affairs in order. Mushtaque, a Pakistani native of Indian descent, was studying chemical engineering at the Indiana Institute of Technology. He immediately contacted his family.

Mushtaque's cousin, a gynecologist, urged Mushtaque's brother to fly him to Los Angeles for treatment at City of Hope National Medical Center, which had just launched its BMT program earlier that year. "My physician . . . was thrilled that I had 10 siblings because it increased the chance for a match," Mushtaque recalled. "I was so fortunate that of my eight siblings tested, all eight matched! My oldest brother, Barkat, who is 14 years my senior, was selected to be the donor after a grueling competition with another brother."

Mushtaque was admitted for a BMT in December 1976. Not surprisingly, he was a bit apprehensive. He knew that none of the first five BMT patients had survived. If he did live through the procedure, he would be City of Hope's first success. "Despite the odds," said Mushtaque, "I was not afraid. I was brought up to believe that we are all born to die, and some go sooner and some go later, so I accepted my situation and moved forward. In retrospect, BMT technology 20 years ago was a bit primitive." For example, patients today receive full-body radiation in short sessions over several days. For Mushtaque, the full-body radiation was delivered in one three-hour, nonstop session after a week of high-dose chemotherapy treatment. "It was like sitting in an oven with the heat on, and the big challenge was keeping me cool," Mushtaque said. "They changed my position every half hour to get all parts of my body. When I left that room, I was actually glowing." The support of the hospital staff and his five siblings, who were constantly at his side throughout the ordeal, made it possible for him to hang on.

For 29 days after the transplantation, Mushtaque was in complete isolation. "At the two-week mark, my doctors tested my bone marrow to see if it had started to make good cells—and it had. I was lucky," he said. Mushtaque also was fortunate that he had minimal graft-versus-host disease and has not had to take any antirejection medications for more than 10 years.

Mushtaque returned to school and studied computer science. Today, he works as a programmer/analyst for a mortgage company. In 1991, he ran in the Los Angeles Marathon. He currently is preparing to ride in a long-distance bike marathon from Los Angeles to San Francisco.

As City of Hope's BMT program celebrates its 20th anniversary, so too does Mushtaque. Not only is he the first person to survive a BMT at City of Hope, but he is the survivor who has lived the longest. "City of Hope is a very special place and an inspiration to all of mankind. It is a miracle garden" Mushtaque said. "I feel it is my second home, and it is always a pleasure to go there. I enjoy speaking to other patients who are undergoing BMT. For them, I am an inspiration." Indeed, Mushtaque is an inspiration to us all.

Lori Baker Schena
Medical writer
California

How do you become a survivor? "You are going to die," two doctors said. First, I got very angry. These guys don't have a crystal ball. They do not know what is going to happen to me. Now, I'll show them a thing or two about how to treat a person with cancer. Over a period of five years, I survived three surgeries, 159 chemotherapy treatments, radiation therapy, and two major hospitalizations—one for blood clots to both lungs and another to have a 3.5-inch piece of broken catheter removed that was floating in my heart. Now, one year later, at age 70, I feel well. The tumor in my liver is not growing. I AM A SURVIVOR of six years!

Charlotte N. Eastley
Wife and mother with colon cancer that spread to her liver
Arizona

Enjoying Life Again

I have learned to be strong and to keep a positive attitude. I accept the fact that not every day will be a good day. It's okay to cry. I always know that tomorrow will be a new day, with new hope. I am enjoying life again.

On Memorial Day weekend 1989, at the age of 34, my family and I vacationed in New Mexico. On our return trip to Lincoln, NE, we were involved in a car accident. The accident alone was a traumatic experience, but the real blow came after the accident. I was advised to immediately see my physician. I underwent computerized tomography scans, x-rays, and other tests. That summer, I had surgery—a left thoracotomy. Surgeons removed my upper left lung lobe because I had cancer. Although the car accident was traumatic, it turned out to be a blessing in disguise.

In 1992, I became very ill. I left work early one day, thinking I had the flu. Three days later, after no improvement, my husband took me to the emergency room, and I was admitted to the intensive care unit for four days. I nearly died. The chaplain and my family members were called under the assumption I would not survive the ordeal. I was diagnosed with Budd Chiari Syndrome, a rare liver disease. My liver was functioning at less than 50%, and doctors told me that I was a potential candidate for a liver transplant. I felt like I had so much life left to live. I did not want to die so young. I wanted to hold my husband. I wanted to be with my family. I was scared and felt totally helpless. I survived, but I spent the next two weeks in the hospital. I will remain on a blood thinner and diuretic for the balance of my life. My blood is monitored monthly, my liver is checked every six months, and I undergo chest x-rays every four months.

In 1994, after four-and-one-half years of chest x-rays, I was really looking forward to living a "normal" life, not attending any more doctor's appointments, missing work, and suffering from the anxiety attacks that preceded the x-rays. That afternoon, I went to my scheduled x-ray and apprehensively awaited the results. I learned that the cancer was back. This time, I had a much more aggressive tumor. I was devastated. Once again, I went through surgery—this time to remove the tumor—followed by four months of chemotherapy, 20 treatments in all. I lost my hair in clumps. I was totally bald. I felt unattractive. I couldn't believe this was happening to me. My husband, family, friends, and coworkers were supportive and tried to humor me through all of the ups and downs. I bought several hats, including baseball caps and a wild hat with a big flower on the front. I even bought a wig, which I never wore. I later donated it to the American Cancer Society. Once again I survived. My friends said, "I can't believe this has happened to you. You're so active."

Then something happened that I would never have imagined. My dear mother was diagnosed with cancer in mid-January 1996. Two weeks after the diagnosis and her second radiation treatment, she passed away. I have adopted a healthier life-style because of the inner strength she had helped me to develop. Three months after her death, I'm Jazzercising five times a week, weight-training four times a week, and eating right. I am stronger and happier, both mentally and physically. I don't think I've ever felt better.

I have loving support from my husband, son, family, and friends. I sometimes feel I can conquer anything and everything. Now I am ready for summer, ready to be with family and friends, ready to go boating and water skiing, and, most importantly, ready to really enjoy life again.

Some days I feel down and depressed. It's then that I am glad I can turn to Jazzercise—for one hour I can concentrate on myself, dance, and let go of all those scary feelings inside. At 41 years "young," I am exercising on a regular basis and enjoying it.

In June 1996, family members, friends, and I formed a team to participate in the American Cancer Society's Relay for Life. This annual event is a 24-hour relay of walking, running, etc. in honor and in memory of patients with cancer and survivors. The donations support cancer research. What a tremendous celebration. This event also enabled me to reestablish bonds with family and friends and to meet new friends and fellow survivors.

I am happy to be here with my husband, my son, my family, and my friends. I would never have made it without them. I have learned to be strong and to keep a positive attitude. I accept the fact that not every day will be a good day and that it is okay to cry. I always know that tomorrow will be a new day with new hope. I am enjoying life again.

Gloria Tune
Cancer survivor
Nebraska

A Race for Life

When I am finished with my chemotherapy, I'm probably going to miss all of that extra attention.

My story started in April of 1994 when I went for my biannual flight physical. My primary physician suggested it would be a good idea to include a sigmoidoscopy. Following this procedure, the doctors discovered a polyp. The doctor said that even though the tumor was benign, it was rather large and was going to have to come out. He wanted to immediately follow-up with a colonoscopy.

At that time, I was training for the Dipsea Race. The Dipsea is the biggest run of the year for runners in Marin County, CA. I have been a runner for more than 25 years and had competed in road races, marathons, and cross-country runs for years. My biggest concern was the disruption a colonoscopy would cause in my training and plans to run the 1994 Dipsea in June. Begrudgingly, the doctor postponed the procedure for six weeks. This would give me enough time to complete my training and run in the Dipsea. I competed, finished 11th, and received a black T-shirt. The coveted numbered black shirts are given to the first 35 runners each year. Many runners, including yours truly, have declared they will be buried in their black shirt.

Five days after the Dipsea, I went to have my colonoscopy. Unfortunately, the doctors felt they couldn't take the tumor out the easy way, so they scheduled me for colon resection surgery the next day. I was a bit in shock. I hadn't been in the hospital since I was a kid having my tonsils out. I have always enjoyed excellent health. Heck, I've been running 2,000 miles a year for the last 20 years—no problems!

I was ready to go home four days after the surgery—a plus that I attribute to the fact that I was in such good shape from running. Then came the real shocker. I was dressed and almost out the door when the doctor told me the tumor was malignant and one of the eight lymph nodes that he took out was cancerous. Based on that, he said I had a year of chemotherapy staring at me.

After the shock wore off and I was able to talk, I learned a lot more about my colon cancer. The love of my life just happens to be an oncology nurse. After she more thoroughly explained the ramifications of what had happened to me and what chemotherapy would be like, I felt a lot better about things. As far as taking or not taking chemotherapy, it was pretty much a no-brainer. I certainly wanted to cut down on my chances of the recurrence of cancer.

When I was lying in the hospital with my black shirt hanging over my bed, my first motivation was that one way or another, I was going to run in the 1995 Dipsea. I was not sure it was going to be possible, but that was going to be my motivation and my goal.

Two weeks after I was released from the hospital, a 10K race we normally run at Kenwood, near Santa Rosa, was being held. I decided my first little goal was to enter that race and walk it—6.2 miles. I was able to walk—not necessarily that comfortably, as I still had lots of aches and pains from my surgery—but I was able to do it. Normally, it takes me 37 minutes to run that race, and it took me about one hour and 30 minutes to walk it.

After that, I started to introduce a little running. The chemotherapy did affect my running. It slowed me down, and I couldn't run my normal six out of seven days a week, which I had been doing for years. I was able, however, to run three or four days weekly, and that was enough to keep me happy.

As far as the side effects of chemotherapy, I really believe the running and exercise helped to move the chemotherapy through my body quickly. I did have many of the various side effects of chemotherapy, but to a mild degree. I had a little bit of nausea, very little. The pills helped. I lost some hair, of course, but because mine is thick, it didn't show very much. It stopped falling out before long and began growing again.

When it came to getting ready for the 1995 Dipsea, I didn't run with my other running friends during hard workouts because I felt I couldn't keep up with them. It was easier for me to do it on my own—on my own schedule and at my own pace.

When Dipsea Day rolled around on June 11, 1995, I cheated a little and skipped my treatment for that week. When the race started, I just told myself to keep on moving and keep thinking, This is the day I am going to beat that cancer. It kept me moving, and, to my great surprise and delight, I finished 23rd overall and received another coveted black shirt. It was a huge emotional victory for me. At the awards ceremony, they gave me the Norman Bright Award, which is an inspirational award presented by 86-year-old Norman Bright, who won the Dipsea back in 1936. He now is legally blind but still comes down for the Dipsea each year to present the award. I was very honored and touched to receive the award.

I recommend anyone undergoing chemotherapy to exercise, which helps physically and psychologically. You don't have to be a running nut like me, but walking, swimming, biking—any aerobic exercise—will definitely help you get through the chemotherapy.

Despite undergoing chemotherapy for a year, I had a lot of fun, and I did a lot of fun things! When I look back on this, I remember the best part of 1995—all of the love and encouragement I received from everybody. When I am finished with my chemotherapy, I'm probably going to miss all of that extra attention.

Stephen P. Lyons
Single male (age 56) with colon cancer
California

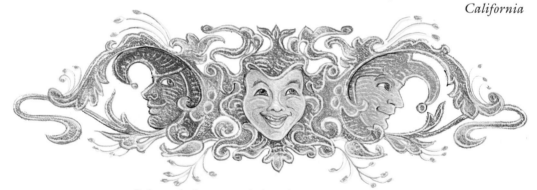

I found that surviving is an ongoing
process that starts the day of diagnosis. It
means to outlive, to live beyond, to keep on
living. My challenge started the day I
began to live life to its fullest each day.

Florence Langer
Fifteen-year survivor of breast cancer
Ohio

The Positive Effects of Cancer

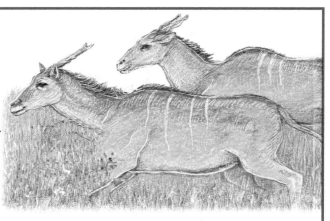

Staying busy sustains a positive effect in that it keeps your mind occupied and can help you forget your problems.

The first positive effect that cancer had on my life focused on changing certain habits in my life-style. I realized that we do not take care of our bodies like we are supposed to. We treat our bodies like they are trash disposals.

Another positive effect was that I became more willing and open about sharing my personal experiences and knowledge about cancer with other people. I believe that people should educate themselves as much as possible so they will not be worried or surprised. If we know what to expect, our fear, anxiety, and, most importantly, ignorance will diminish. Even though we know that we should get second opinions, we often are hesitant because we do not want to offend our physicians. When we discuss cancer with others, we must realize that obtaining a second opinion is not only our right but also something that could save our lives.

The most important way that cancer has affected my life is my renewed sense of faith and a more positive attitude. I am a firm believer in "mind over matter." Staying busy sustains a positive effect in that it keeps your mind occupied and can help you forget your problems. In my case, even though I can retire, I continue working every day. I believe that if I stayed home, I would make myself sick from worrying about every little thing.

Ramiro Rosales
Pharyngeal cancer survivor
as interviewed by Guadalupe Palos, LMSW, RN,
cancer nurse and niece of Ramiro Rosales
Texas

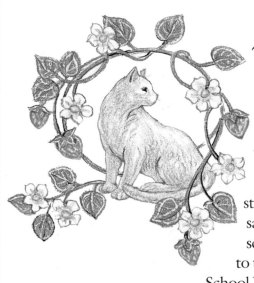

Welcome Back

All of these amazing people helped me to keep a positive attitude—which is a must. I feel certain that attitude is half of the battle.

"We would like to welcome back a former staff member who has been given a new life," said Mr. McKelvey, the principal of one of my schools, as he introduced new staff members to the 250-plus members of the Gallipolis City School District.

"Several years ago, our school nurse found herself facing an illness that had literally stricken her overnight. She awoke to find herself in a face-to-face battle with leukemia. Today, she is living proof that miracles still happen. Through God's grace, many prayers, her own faith, and the help of doctors, nurses, and modern medicine, she escaped death in overcoming this battle."

I couldn't believe it! I knew that I would be introduced with the new staff, but this was incredible! I heard the emotion in Mr. McKelvey's voice, and I was in tears as he continued.

"It was the will to live for her family and friends that has allowed her to be back with us today. No one (in our district) has ever returned to work from disability leave before, so this is a first for me. By now, I'm sure you know whom I'm talking about. We would like to welcome back our school nurse, Cathy Elliott."

I was so touched by this speech that I ended up crying in a big way. As I stood, so did the entire staff—and they applauded! I felt as if I would burst with joy! What a miracle! Four years ago I was preparing to die, and now, here I am—back to work!

My uphill battle started in May of 1992. I experienced flu-like symptoms that I couldn't shake. I was in a local hospital for three days and then was sent to the Ohio State University's James Cancer Hospital and Research Institute.

During the next 44 days of hospitalization, I was diagnosed with acute lymphocytic leukemia (ALL), and my prognosis was not very good.

My illness had forced me to abandon my family. My eight-year-old daughter, Bethany, and five-year-old-son, Matthew, didn't know what to think as they were shuffled from relative to relative.

Steve, my husband, was torn between his sick wife, his children, and his job. He took every Wednesday off work to drive the two hours to Columbus to be with me. He also spent every weekend at my bedside. When he couldn't be there, he arranged for family and friends to visit me on alternating days so I wouldn't be alone. Steve's love and devotion still amaze me!

I knew that God was with me from the very beginning. I can remember telling my parents, "It's going to be all right." I was at peace with whatever was going to happen. I was literally half-dead and dazed when I made that statement. Later, as I realized the severity of my disease, my faith did waver a bit. I cried as I never cried before.

The love and support of my family and friends over the next 16 months of treatments gave me the strength and courage to face each day. Everyone pitched in to make our lives as normal as possible. All of these amazing people helped me to keep a positive attitude—which is a must. I feel certain that attitude is half of the battle. The rest of the battle is won through God's grace. After all, God gave my doctors and nurses the knowledge they needed to help save my life. God showed my family's needs to people who helped to meet those needs. God walks beside me every day.

After being so very ill and near death's door, I feel that I should have something very profound to say, something that will help people in a similar situation, something that will heal, but all I know to say is this: God is real, and He is still in the business of saving lives and souls.

Cathy Elliott, RN, BSPA
Acute lymphocytic leukemia survivor of four-and-one-half years
Ohio

The most fascinating part of an illness, to me, is the part that's seldom discussed—the healing. Like a work of art or life itself, the healing processes move out from under your well-meant intentions and go where they please.

Lora Wise McKenna
Cancer survivor
Pennsylvania

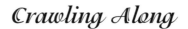

Crawling Along

Oh, to once again
Feel the breeze blow through my hair.
A common thing to others
Is a cancer patient's prayer.

What do you expect from me?
I'm trying to endure.
What is there left for me?
I really can't be sure.

So, I've decided to fight for life
In spite of what I've lost.
I'll never give up, never give out—
No matter what the cost.

I'll look in my mirror each morning,
and if a reflection is there,
I'll thank you for all that is left,
And praise you with my prayer.

I'll thank you for my children,
Who have suffered so much, too.
I'll thank you for their love,
And all they helped me do.

I can say so many thanks
For all my faithful friends,
Who stood by me through the fearful days
When life was near the end.

And, God, I could never say enough,
Not in a million years,
For the doctors and the nurses
Who cared for me and helped me bear my fears.

God, be with your cancer patients,
To help them to endure,
Until we hear the magic words . . .
"At last! We've found a Cure!"

Barbara Burney
After a four-year battle, she succumbed to ovarian cancer
Submitted by Monte Wise, RN, BSN, OCN®
Texas

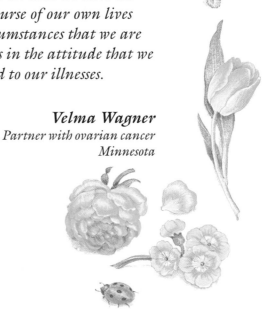

I read somewhere that you can't change the direction of the wind, but you can adjust your sails. It reminds me that we have the power to chart the course of our own lives regardless of the circumstances that we are dealt. Healing comes in the attitude that we bring to our lives and to our illnesses.

Velma Wagner
Partner with ovarian cancer
Minnesota

What Did I Have to Fear?

I was determined that I would keep my sense of humor, even though I had lost my voice.

I started smoking at the age of 14 while at school in England. I smoked my way around the world as a member of the Royal Navy, and I smoked my way to America as an immigrant in 1987.

I developed a hoarse voice soon after my arrival in this country, but I attributed it to air conditioning or allergies—anything but a smoking-related condition. On my 50th birthday, in 1990, my doctor informed me that my recent biopsy showed a malignant tumor of the larynx.

I was hastily referred to the Medical College of Virginia in Richmond. The doctors decided that a course of radiation therapy would cure the problem. Thirty-two doses of radiation later, the tumor was gone. Soon after that, I started smoking again. After all, I had beaten cancer once. What did I have to fear?

Two years later, on October 22, 1992, I had difficulty breathing and swallowing. My wife was at work that evening, and my discomfort was so acute that I decided to call 911. The paramedics found me unconscious in the doorway of our home. The cancer had suddenly returned—worse than before. I was rushed to the hospital, where my own ear, nose, and throat doctor was on call. He immediately informed me that my breathing difficulty could be eased by performing a tracheostomy, but I couldn't have a general anesthetic. The surgery was extremely painful, even with a local anesthetic, because the radiation therapy had not only shrunk the previous tumor but had scarred the trachea.

I was transported back to Richmond, where the doctors decided that surgical removal of the larynx was my only option. I underwent that surgery on Friday, November 13, 1992.

I was determined that I would keep my sense of humor even though I had lost my voice. Immediately after my surgery, I was being fed liquid nutritional supplements through a tube that passed up my nose and straight down to my stomach (bypassing my taste buds). I asked one of the nurses if I could please have strawberry or chocolate because I did not like the vanilla—and she complied!

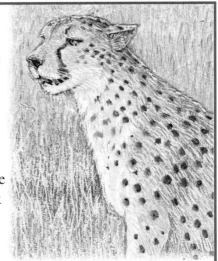

I now speak using an electro larynx, a device that makes me sound like a computer. I speak to groups of school children on the dangers and consequences of smoking, not only for themselves but also for their loved ones.

My electro larynx really gets their attention. It is a wonderful tool in my motivational speeches. After all, they can hear this consequence and not just imagine it.

Frank Morgan
Four-year laryngectomee
Virginia

Keeping busy made me feel safer, but there was a constant battle going on inside me. I was having a hard time doing what Rilke described as "walking side by side with the beast." I tried hiding, but that didn't work. Friends or relatives wrote or spoke to me by phone, and I was immersed in love. Each voice became a lily pad that held me up while I traversed mysterious waters.

Lora Wise McKenna
Cancer survivor
Pennsylvania

To Live or to Die?

"I'm not going to let someone cut me open, go through that pain, and then die anyway."

He lay in the hospital bed, stern-faced, angry, and adamant in his decision. He'd just been told that he had renal cancer and that surgery was his best shot at survival. He was determined to refuse any operation. "I'm not going to let someone cut me open, go through that pain, and then die anyway. I'll just get a cyanide pill and finish it off now."

Maury was an ex-Marine who'd survived Guadalcanal. He was now in his late 70s, still as tough as he was then, and not about to let himself suffer. As I sat with him, he told me of his intention to end his life quickly. He obviously was a practical man, so I tried to keep my arguments logical.

Suppose you kill yourself today, not knowing whether your cancer is curable by surgery. What would it hurt to think it over, get a second opinion, maybe have the surgery, and then see how things look? You can always kill yourself later if that's what you really want. But if you do it now, you eliminate all other choices. And what about the feelings of your family? He reluctantly agreed to think it over.

I saw him a few weeks later—postoperatively. He was cranky because of pain but smiling because the news was good. He was chafing to get out of the hospital and back home with his wife.

It was two years before I saw him again. He came by the unit to say hello and thanks—fresh from a visit to the doctor. He grinned all over as he told me that his checkup showed no recurrence. He felt great!

Recently, I kept my promise to stop by his home. I found him, at 79 years old, standing on a ladder washing windows. He and his wife welcomed me. They proudly showed me around their yard, sharing goodies from the garden and stories from their lives— especially the last two years.

Thelma Hulka, RN, OCN®
Oncology nurse
Illinois

If someone mentions cancer
It scares me half to death!
And if ice is placed upon my back
It will surely take my breath;
But in time the ice will melt away
and I hope my cancer does the same.

Dave Kekar
Throat cancer survivor
Indiana

Nancy and I found something to laugh at
every day. It helped us get through the
worst times and elevated us from the
seriousness of cancer. Bill Cosby's statement,
"If you can laugh at it, you can
survive it," was true for us.

Velma Wagner
Partner with ovarian cancer
Minnesota

After surgery for prostate
cancer at the ripe old age of
42, I was told I only had three
years to live. To confirm this,
the hospital chaplain read me
my last rites. But this didn't
scare me. I was already scared
to death—too scared to enter the
hospital chapel down the hall
during my walks. Now,
three years later, I'm still in
remission!

Tom Bassett
Prostate cancer survivor
Vermont

Two Miracle Patients

"I am glad my doctors were better at treating cancer than they were at forecasting my future!"

Miracle One: I met Lucy about a year-and-a-half ago at a cancer support group for women with breast or gynecological cancers. We started the meeting by going around the room and introducing ourselves. Lucy's presence filled the room as she spoke. In a very calm, steady voice, she explained that she recently had been diagnosed with stage IV cervical cancer and her chances for survival were very poor. "I am terminal," she said.

The room fell silent for a moment, but my mind was screaming, "No!" I wanted to shout, "You are not terminal!" It was physically difficult for me to remain in my chair because I wanted to leap across the room, hug Lucy, and tell her that her doctor was wrong. I had been an oncology nurse for 15 years, and this was not denial or naivete on my part. I simply *knew* that Lucy would survive.

As the weeks went by and the support group continued to meet, Lucy shared her feelings about her treatment and side effects, in addition to her hopes and feelings about being "terminal." I always was struck by how full of life Lucy was! Her smooth skin glowed. She had an angelic way of reaching out to other group members—she exuded a positive, radiant sense of serenity, and I enjoyed being in her presence.

About a year later, Lucy heard those three precious letters that are music to the ears: Lucy was declared "NED" (no evidence of disease). She now spends her time enjoying water aerobics and her farm instead of attending chemotherapy appointments. I enjoy carrying her inspirational story in my heart.

Miracle Two: I regularly refer to Dean as "Miracle Man." Dean and I also met at a cancer support group in 1987. Nearly two years earlier, Dean had been treated with radiation therapy for inoperable lung cancer. I was surprised by this news. In 1985, it was unusual for patients to survive with that diagnosis. In fact, until that point, Dean was the first survivor I had met! Dean was very inspirational to the group, with his tales of golfing, walking to radiation appointments, and even riding his stationary bike 25 miles a day after having been told that he was terminal.

Three years after his initial diagnosis, his doctor discovered that Dean had metastasis to the brain. Dean underwent whole-brain radiation. I was certain that we would lose him from our support group. I love being wrong about these things! More than 10 years after his initial diagnosis, Dean continues to be an inspiration to many people. As he likes to say, "I am glad my doctors were better at treating cancer than they were at forecasting my future!"

Mary Gerbracht, RN, MSN, AOCN
Oncology nurse, formerly of Dallas, TX
California

Eric, an athlete who was diagnosed with leukemia, taught me about courage and about the importance of hope. Incurability is a state of the body; hopelessness is a state of mind. Patients can tolerate incurability, but not hopelessness.

Barbara Livingston, RN, OCN®
Oncology nurse
New Jersey

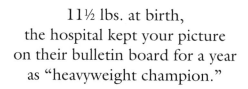

Neil: The Heavyweight Champion

11½ lbs. at birth,
the hospital kept your picture
on their bulletin board for a year
as "heavyweight champion."

2½ years old,
I discovered bruises
up and down your legs.
"My God," I pondered,
"What is this?"

Doctors' diagnosis . . .
Leukemia—
Cancer in your blood.
A part of your dad and me
died that day.

My daily life became
a blur.
Giving you medicine each morning,
I grew numb to fear and pain.

Finding blonde clumps of hair
on your pillow one morning,
I wept and wept.
You didn't understand
my shedding of tears.

I lay prostrate before God,
over and over
begging mercy for your life
and asking strength
to take you to the hospital
for your treatments.

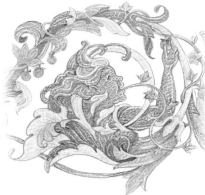

Paul, a little older than you,
(With such a kind smile)
died.
He also had leukemia and
he caught pneumonia.

Deep grief and sorrow—
for Paul and his family—
overcame me.
Again I was faced with
the seriousness of your condition.

Buoyed up by all the prayers
of family and friends,
hours, minutes, days, weeks, and seasons
all became one, long journey.

Final biopsy...
"All clear," the doctor said, "All clear."
Neil, in that one short moment of time,
the relief your dad and I experienced
will take an eternity for you to know.
We wept, we laughed, we praised,
we thanked, we let go of you
and you were given back to us.
Thanks be to God.

Debbie Bradshaw
Mother of 14-year-old son, Neil,
who was diagnosed at age 2½ with leukemia
Ohio

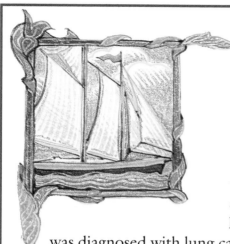

When Life Stood Still

Cliff knew that his father was now his "guardian angel."

Some time ago, I received a precious gift in the form of my husband, Cliff. Our life stood still in 1994 when he was diagnosed with lymphoma—only one month after his father was diagnosed with lung cancer. To add insult to injury, he had a surgical biopsy performed on his 48th birthday!

Together, father and son embarked on a journey through chemotherapy, supporting each other every step of the way. Sadly, his father lost his battle. Cliff continued his treatment, focusing on his father's strength and knowing that his father was now his "guardian angel" who guided him from above. Since his goal of complete remission was not to be, the only alternative for a cure was a bone marrow transplant. Cliff is such a caring, giving person that he decided to tape record the entire bone marrow transplant process in the hope that it could help someone else. We also took daily pictures, and, believe me, a picture is definitely worth a thousand words. This was *his* form of therapy. It helped to keep him focused and maintain his ever-present positive attitude.

Cliff volunteers at the Cleveland Clinic to share his experience with patients with lymphoma who are about to undergo bone marrow transplant. When he receives a request, he telephones the patient prior to admission and follows up with calls throughout their hospitalization. Then he surprises them with a visit. Their goal is to go home in fewer days and, invariably, one of their first phone calls once they get home is to let Cliff know they are home and well. What a good feeling that is!

To celebrate Cliff's first birthday following his bone marrow transplant, we took a cruise on the newest "Love Boat." We also renewed our marriage vows while on board. It was a most memorable cruise. Something amazing happened while the crew was singing "Happy Birthday" to Cliff. A male passenger whom we had just met came to our table, shook Cliff's hand, and, unexpectantly, kissed him on the cheek! It turned out that his wife was also a cancer survivor, and he was caught up in our "Celebration of Life." After that, several more people came over to relate their own success stories. It was so heartwarming!

It is now nearly two years later, and so far, so good! I love and appreciate my husband, Clifford Hilliard Wedge, more and more with each passing day!

Donna Wedge
Proud wife of a two-year bone marrow transplant survivor
Ohio

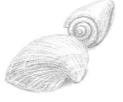

The entire experience changed my life. Though I hated the suffering I had to endure, I'm stronger because of it.

Judy Gmetro
Five-year ovarian cancer survivor
Illinois

We need to keep physically and spiritually fit. Standing on top of the snow-capped Alps in Austria, I felt closer to my higher power—so close I didn't want to come down.

Tom Bassett
Prostate cancer survivor
Vermont

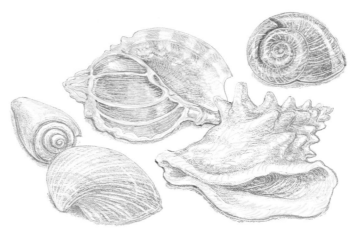

When Time Stands Still: Is It Cancer?

Aren't I glorious? I'm alive! I'm alive!

Routine blood test.
The doctor's pace, manner, and tone abruptly change:
Your blood count is suddenly
Ten times normal;
We suspect leukemia.
Your lung x-ray has a suspicious shadow;
We recommend a CT scan
To check for a malignant tumor.
Get these tests right away.
More tests, still more tests . . .
Come back next Monday.

I stand alone.
Stunned,
Confused,
Overwhelmed
As the doctor's secretary hands me
So many papers
Test orders, directions
The world slips into slow motion . . .
Her words float by me
Like cotton candy in my brain
Sticky, puffy
Too much to swallow.

Time shifts to a surrealistic quality.
I'm surprised how normal
How calm my voice sounds,
But my words seem to come
From someone else
Suddenly separate from me
As I slip out of my body
And watch myself
As if from a distance.
The space between filled with

Dull numbness
Covering a chilling fear
Pushing down a growing panic.

Later at home
I call friends for support.
No answer.
No one is home.
Errands and kitchen piles
Seem insurmountable, irrelevant.
I go out
Destination somewhere,
Anywhere away.
Where can I run away?

I escape to the park garden.
Sensational rainbow cascade of
Lush shimmering summer flowers
Jolts me back into the present.
Intense racy red feathery plumes
Swish gently on my soul.
Thick green strong stalks of
Giant golden spectacular sunflowers,
Proud beaming broad faces
Towering six feet high
Draw my energy upward with wonder.
Lacy luscious globes of hot pink petals
Burst like a furious flurry of
Fantastic fireworks
Exploding effervescently,
Exhilarating my heart
With a resounding but unheard
Life-affirming boom.
God's palette spills out in such
Awesome abundance.

Magnificent monarch butterfly
Flutters gracefully from blossom to blossom
Pauses so near, just a few inches away
Expansive six-inch-wide lacy wings
Intricately etched
By an unseen divine artist
Silently shouts
Wake up!
Pay attention!
Notice me!
Aren't I glorious?
I'm alive! I'm alive!

Betsy Firger
Attorney, wife, and mother of three teenagers and
four-year survivor of non-Hodgkin's lymphoma
Connecticut

I learned many things from this experience. The most important was to learn to deal with stress in a less destructive fashion. Now, when something is less than desirable in my life, I tackle it right away. I do not let it fester inside of me. I try to be more patient. It is easy to say "I understand," but I have learned that unless you have experienced cancer yourself, you cannot understand the flight of emotions.

Kathie Gepfert, RN
One-year breast cancer survivor
Colorado

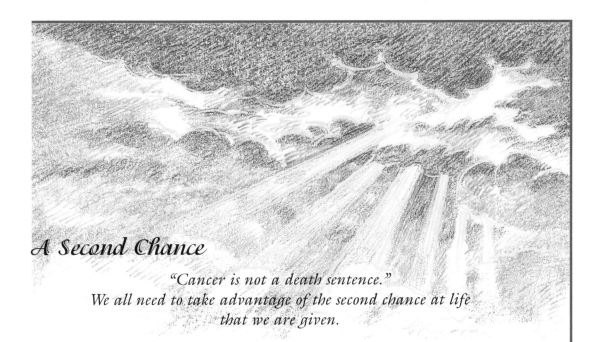

A Second Chance

"Cancer is not a death sentence."
We all need to take advantage of the second chance at life
that we are given.

I started smoking when I was 12 years old. I was a two-pack-a-day smoker for more than 30 years. In 1984, I lost my voice and was treated for laryngitis. By 1987, I wanted a second opinion. I was then diagnosed with throat cancer. In 1988, the surgery to remove my cancer also removed my voice box. I was devastated. I also had an infection in my lymph nodes, which could have led to my death. To make the situation even worse, my marriage fell apart, and I was left to take care of my son, Dwayne, alone. I felt abandoned. I was forced to leave my job. My income was depleted from my ex-wife's drug habit. I was on disability for one-and-one-half years. Everything I had worked for was gone and could not be replaced.

Somehow I made it! I began to help rehabilitate other people with laryngectomies. I became the president of a large support group. I created a workshop with the help of other members. I now volunteer for the American Cancer Society to educate school children on the dangers of tobacco use. I urge them to quit or never start smoking. I also work as a volunteer with the state of California to promote tobacco education for people of all ages. I am a facilitator for "I Quit" and "Fresh Start" smoking cessation classes. I also work with hospitals and companies to educate patients with laryngectomies on the latest surgical procedures and devices. I support the American Heart Association, American Lung Association, and National Cancer Institute in their lawsuit against the tobacco industry. It will never replace what I have lost, but I hope it can help prevent harm to others.

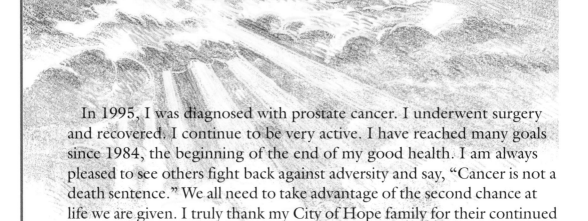

In 1995, I was diagnosed with prostate cancer. I underwent surgery and recovered. I continue to be very active. I have reached many goals since 1984, the beginning of the end of my good health. I am always pleased to see others fight back against adversity and say, "Cancer is not a death sentence." We all need to take advantage of the second chance at life we are given. I truly thank my City of Hope family for their continued support and encouragement.

Lou Bolduc
Throat and prostate cancer survivor
California

My advice to the newly diagnosed is to face your disease head on. Pray, keep the faith, and don't give up hope. Don't ever quit fighting. Savor every day of your life. Develop an appreciation of the true value life contains and put things in perspective— where life, love, and people are ever more important than money or material possessions. Develop a positive and philosophical attitude about life—and about death. Do the very best you can to conquer your disease. Live one day at a time, accepting whatever the future holds for you. Fear is useless. What is needed is trust.

Stanley F. Stefanski
Survivor of urinary and colon cancer with liver metastasis
Illinois

Don't Stay in the Basement

In 1992, Karen received a diagnosis of metastatic ovarian cancer. She was told she had a one in three chance of surviving three years. Her approach in coping with her cancer was to face it with optimism. Karen recognized that cancer affects so many more people than just the patient. Families also feel frustration and a sense of powerlessness. Her husband, Stan, told her to quit working and enjoy the time she had left. At age 47, Karen stated, "A whole new light was cast on my life. From then on I enjoyed everything I could—even my chemotherapy!" When she lost her hair following chemotherapy treatment, her young daughter, Ashley, worried that her mom's hair would come in bright red. Now, four years later, Ashley is using a strawberry rinse on her own hair! How things change!

"There are positive things about cancer," she explained. "It makes you realize what is important and what isn't." During her chemotherapy treatments, she began to plan for things that were important to her, such as arranging family trips and redecorating her daughter's bedroom. Karen feels most grateful that she has been able to watch and enjoy their daughter Ashley move through the transition years from 8 to 12.

Four years later and cancer-free, Karen said she felt like the "luckiest person alive" and wanted to give other patients with cancer hope. She now does this on a weekly basis as a volunteer on the oncology unit of Memorial Medical Center in Springfield, IL. As she moves in and out of patient rooms, delivering mail and refilling water pitchers, she carries cheer and a potent message, "Never let cancer stop you!" She tells patients and families, "It is okay to feel depressed, but don't stay in the basement. Enjoy every day and save your energy for the things you really want to do."

Karen follows her own advice on this. She always wanted to drive her husband's Harley. Now she has her motorcycle licence and her own Honda Ace Bike. "I would never have driven a bike before I had cancer, but after facing cancer, riding a bike is just not so scary anymore!"

Sue Dinges, RN
Staff nurse on an oncology unit
Illinois

How Sweet This Perspective Is!

"There is never enough time to do or say all the things we would wish. The thing is to try to do as much as you can with the time that you have. Time is short and suddenly you're not there any more."
—From *A Christmas Carol,* by Charles Dickens

CRISIS: On August 18, 1987, I pulled up in my driveway to see my doctor sitting on my front porch swing. I plopped down beside him, puzzled by his presence. He then began a stream of tenderly spoken words that kicked me sharply in the face. Dazed, I managed to eke out, "Thank you for coming here to tell me."

More words followed, but I wasn't there for them. I was drowning in the echo of the "C" word—*cancer.* Finally, I said, "Is there a cure?"

"I don't know."

"How long do I have to live?"

"Let's step inside." We did. He took my hands in his, looked me straight in the eye, and said, "I don't know how long you have to live."

HEARTBREAK: Then the tidal wave of tears began. First me, then Cal, Mom and Dad, my family, and my friends. We had to cry together. Then we had to cry separately—in closets, bathrooms, wherever and whatever hour we could find privacy. Pain, shock, denial, anger, negotiation, despair, acceptance—I've felt it all. There was a phase of "Why me? It's not fair. I've led a basically good life. I just don't deserve this. I have a husband and a one- and a four-year-old. They need me. The whole thing stinks!"

PERSEVERANCE: Amid all this chaos, friends and family kept saying, "You can fight this thing and beat it." But *cancer* seemed so frightening and overpowering. The word still stuck in my throat. There I was at rock bottom, feeling *so* sorry for myself, when I realized I had a choice: bite the bullet or bite the dust. I recall that as a child I had broken my leg while horseback riding. After hospitalization, complications, a wheelchair, and crutches, my parents taught me it was critical to get back on the horse and face my fears. Before giving in to it all, I decided to negotiate the situation. I was back in the saddle again.

Then I did what any other self-respecting, obsessive-compulsive, Type A personality would do. I devised a strategic battle plan for conquering "the monster within." I worked from the premise if it can't hurt you and it might help, go for it.

That's when the tragedy stopped and the adventure began.

ADVENTURE: I read everything I could get my hands on. I knew that treatment was life-threatening in itself; the initial odds I received were a 50% chance to survive the bone marrow transplant procedure. Since patients who receive transplants within a year of diagnosis have a better prognosis, I decided to take interferon for 10 months and then go ahead with it.

I crammed 40 years of living into those 10 months. First, I focused on family and friends—my social side. I vacationed in Mexico with them, went to Disney World with Cal and our children, reunited with longtime buddies, and enjoyed a "hugging party." I laughed until my sides ached, cried until my eyes swelled, and spoke tender words that are too often left unsaid. I shared agonies, ecstasies, and coping techniques with other patients with cancer at Baylor's self-help support group. I understand why someone once observed, "No one on his deathbed ever said, 'I wish I'd spent more time on my business.'" Loved ones are everything.

Besides all the relating, I ate my fill of healthy food, got ample sleep, exercised with Jane Fonda, and listened to visualization, imaging, and relaxation tapes.

Conquering my mind was another challenge. I broke my strategy down into four areas:

Interpretation: It's not just what's happening to me, it's how I interpret and respond to it. Do I have a 50% chance of disaster or a 50% chance to live?

Control: I studied all the options I *did* have and prioritized.

Positive self-talk: I acknowledged my negative thoughts and then tried to replace them with optimistic, constructive, yet realistic ones.

Sense of purpose: Like Alice in Wonderland, if you don't know where you're going, you'll probably end up someplace else. I reaffirmed worthwhile goals: have fun, help others, learn something new, and emphasize motherhood. I developed courage, guts, grit, nerve, gumption, chutzpah, and intestinal fortitude. It's the belief that you can do what you feel you can't do.

Finally, I dealt with my spiritual side. Someone said, "There are no atheists in foxholes." When facing a crisis, it's natural to do some philosophical and theological soul-searching. Though there were no easy answers to my questions, by reaffirming my faith, I derived intense comfort from a strong sense of being cradled in God's everlasting arms during some of my most terrifying moments.

Before I left for the transplant facility in Seattle, I spent a beautiful weekend in Galveston with Cal and the children, which included mud fights on the beach and heartbreaking embraces as we parted. The kids went to Abilene to visit my in-laws while Cal spent six weeks of the most critical period with me. My donor brother Bubba stayed a month; my parents were there the entire four months.

I stayed afloat by attempting my coping strategies and enjoying personal visits, cards, letters, phone calls, touching gifts, and wacky gimmicks initiated by friends. One of these was a 4 x 6-foot colossalgram proclaiming "Even bald, Texas women are beautiful." I resorted to a few zany antics myself. One day I put up a poster in my window facing the street that read, "Help! I'm a prisoner in a laminar airflow unit!"

PERSPECTIVE: Today, one year after my transplant, I've resumed a new normal life. I've had to call on strengths that I didn't know I had. Now there is more empathy, openness, honesty, contentment, toughness, and perspective. I've learned that life is fragile. But in spite of the pain and the buckets of tears that were shed, my cancer crisis has been one of the most enriching experiences of my life. I am now more fully aware and appreciative of the full gamut of life, and I've found new dimensions in myself.

I savor and cherish every moment. I smell the grass when I cut it, bask in the feel of the sun on my face, and watch ants and clouds go by. I actually enjoy driving in a car pool and even revel in the earsplitting cacophony of my kids' occasional tantrums—all priceless events, precious gifts of wonder. Life is now more three-dimensional, and as the artist Uccello exclaimed, "Oh, what a sweet thing this perspective is!"

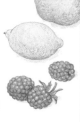

Now more than ever, I heed Dickens' admonition from *A Christmas Carol*: "There is never enough time to do or say all the things we would wish. The thing is to try to do as much as you can with the time that you have. Time is short and suddenly you're not there any more."

Clare Buie Chaney, PhD
Licensed professional counselor and 10-year leukemia survivor
Texas

It was a day we would never forget. It was a picture-perfect fall day. The sky was clear, the sun was shining, and the leaves were changing from summer green to beautiful autumn colors. Little did we realize, our lives, like the autumn leaves, would soon change as well.

Sheila Becker
Mother of son with
brain cancer (5½-year survivor)
Ohio

Losing my hair was the worst part of having cancer. It bothered me to admit this. I mean, what kind of a shallow person would worry about losing her hair when she had a serious disease? Meeting Roberta, who was diagnosed with cancer at age 24, was a blessing for me. She helped me put my hair loss in perspective.

Rosemary Umbriac
Ovarian cancer survivor
Pennsylvania

Roots and Records

Video and audio taping, especially of older family members, is a wonderful way to employ modern technology to preserve family legends, lore, and maybe a few lives.

Cancer was discovered in my left breast in 1975. I have fought this disease with all my personal strength. It often took an incredible force of will on my part just to get up in the morning, let alone go on with life—but I did. I want to share one aspect of many messages of optimism and joy I discovered through this experience.

I believe that a strong sense of self is derived from knowledge of our roots. The study of our origins and personal history provides a way to examine and test the ingrained patterns and ideas that have prevailed for centuries. Everyone should keep some kind of record of life's occurrences. I do this by compiling scrapbooks.

My husband is an amateur photographer and provides the material for a fine visual history. I save and collect odd items of memorabilia that further enhance the picture story. Among other things, I saved our children's report cards, Mother's Day cards, baby teeth, letters of explanation after a misunderstanding, unexpected thank-you messages, and invitations. Together, we have created a pictorial and written chronicle for every year of our life. Our joint effort to hand down a historical record to our children is just one small way of keeping our intimate relationship current.

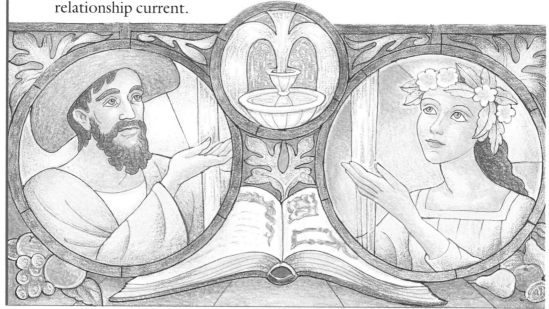

Other ways to document the past include keeping a written journal or arranging old letters in chronological order. Video and audio taping, especially of older family members, also is a wonderful way to employ modern technology to preserve family legends, lore, and maybe a few lives. Whatever form the record-keeping takes, it is essential that it be kept for future generations. These projects helped me as I traveled the journey to recovery.

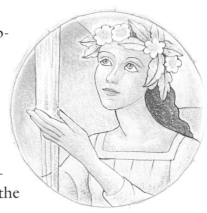

Rena J. Blumberg
Breast cancer survivor
Ohio

My Mom is my hero. She has shown me how to fight things, stay tough, and never give up. I didn't know how strong she was until she faced breast cancer. It always seemed the chances were low for her to make it, but she kept proving the odds wrong. When the chemotherapy did not solve the cancer, the next choice was death—with no hope—or a very dangerous bone marrow transplant. I remember the first day that I came to see her in the hospital after she'd had the transplant. She didn't even look like my Mom—more like a baboon. She ended up making it out of there in 21 days, which was the hospital record. The cancer was all gone. Now I know never to give up. Always believe in yourself.

Ted Kerr
Ninth-grader and son of mother with breast cancer
Ohio

Slaying Dragons

You need only arm yourself with perseverance, empowering thoughts, loved ones, and laughter and cradle yourself in the love of your God . . . and oh, what an adventure life will be!

I would like to share the words I have gleaned from others regarding things that helped get me through my cancer experience.

1. **Perseverance:** In Texan terms, I was going to "take the bull by the horns." I had to give it my best shot, so I decided that "a mommy's gotta do what a mommy's gotta do." I adopted Winston Churchill's World War II battle cry, "Never, never, *never*, give up."

2. **Empowering thoughts:** "The real voyage of discovery consists not in seeking new lands but in seeing with new eyes" (Marcel Proust). Though I couldn't change the direction of the wind, I *could* adjust my sails. As my oncology nurse put it, "We are all faced with a series of great opportunities, *brilliantly* disguised as impossible situations." Through my counseling training, I had learned to reinterpret negative, fearful thoughts into positive, constructive ones. My transplant offered me a 50/50 chance to *live;* the cup was not half empty, it was half full. I realized I *could* do what I *felt* I couldn't—I could feel the fear and yet do it anyway.

3. **Loved ones:** Two-year-old Clark's first uttered sentence was one of encouragement: "Don't worry, Mommy." My husband, Cal's favorite motivator was the Nike phrase: "Just do it!" A friend said, "Clare, you can bloom where you're planted." My psychiatrist father's comforting remark was, "Clare, it's normal to feel crazy right now. You'd be crazy to feel normal!" My mother supplied her comforting philosophy on housework not getting done: "Clare, if you don't eat off it, why clean it?"

4. **Laughter:** "She who laughs, lasts." In some pretty pitiful moments, I donned my Carmen Miranda fruit turban and learned to laugh at myself. Some favorite punch lines were "Calgon, take me away!" "Goof and grow!" "It could've been worse!" "Life is good, life is good . . ." "We are but tiny bugs on the windshield of life." "Yard by

yard, it's too hard; inch by inch, it's a cinch!" "This, too, shall pass."
Assigning a number to a cuss word and yelling: "Number five!"

5. **Faith:** It is best summed up by a child in Sunday school class who said, "God's hands are *so* big, you can never fall out of them!" Feeling cradled in God's loving arms got me through some of my loneliest, most terrifying moments.

Only in fairy tales does the hero slay the dragon and live happily ever after. In real life, the dragons—the obstacles, the challenges—keep coming. Just remember that these seemingly impossible situations are merely brilliantly disguised *great* opportunities; you need only arm yourself with perseverance, empowering thoughts, loved ones, and laughter as you cradle yourself in the love of your God . . . and, oh, what an adventure it will be!

Clare Buie Chaney, PhD
Licensed professional counselor and 10-year leukemia survivor
Texas

The day I was scheduled for bilateral mastectomies arrived. I suddenly realized that this previously dreaded surgery was the miracle that would save my life! The surgery became my friend, my lifesaver, my miracle, and my epiphany. I now welcomed it.

Nancy Gilbert Phillips
Breast cancer survivor
Arizona

Once a person begins a trip through the cancer experience, he or she is likely to encounter some unexpected turns. The traveler may need to take on a different role with each new bend in the road.

Joanne Hindle, RN, BSN, OCN®
Cancer survivor, oncology nurse, and daughter of cancer survivor
Colorado

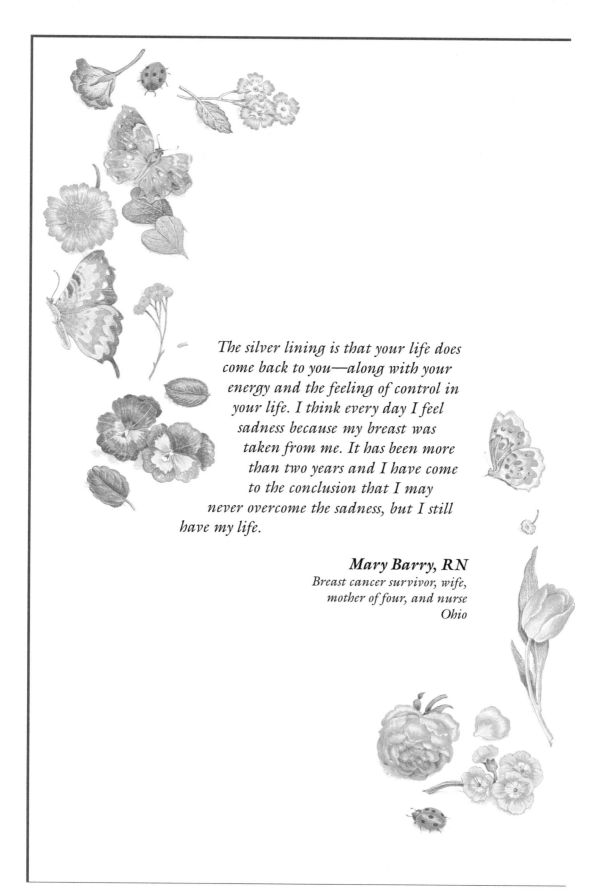

The silver lining is that your life does come back to you—along with your energy and the feeling of control in your life. I think every day I feel sadness because my breast was taken from me. It has been more than two years and I have come to the conclusion that I may never overcome the sadness, but I still have my life.

Mary Barry, RN
Breast cancer survivor, wife,
mother of four, and nurse
Ohio

Chapter 2

Love: The Best Umbrella

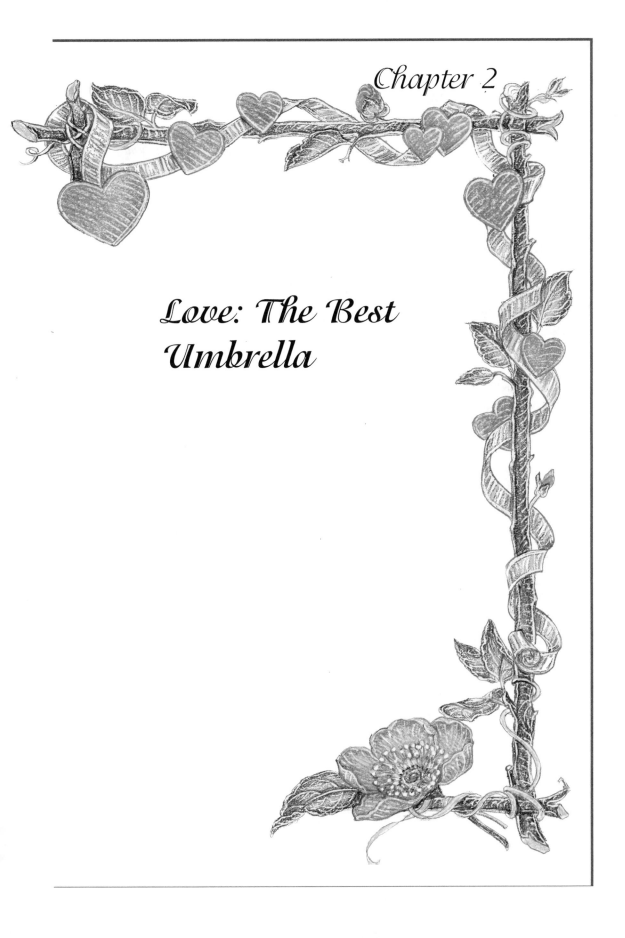

Twelve Roses

She survived using the kind of heroism shown only to those who watch and wait. I was there for her. I will always be there for her.

Every year on a day in October, I visit a flower shop and buy a dozen roses. It is not my wife's birthday, our anniversary, or because I forgot to do something. This day marks the time we learned she had breast cancer. That day lives in my mind as a nightmare of lost hope, mortal despair, and holding hands in the dark. Besides dealing with our own fears of cancer, we also needed to tell our 12-year-old son the bad news.

I remember her struggle to cling to this fragile life. She once told me, "I do not want to be forgotten." She survived using the kind of heroism shown only to those who watch and wait. I was there for her. I will always be there for her.

I continue to buy roses every October. My son, who is aware of this ritual, playfully criticized, "You're not doing that again, are you, Dad?"

"This day is important," I explained to him. "Each year your mother survives, I add one pink rose to replace the white ones. White roses are like uncolored canvases resembling hope for other pink roses to complete the dozen."

My son placed the roses into a vase after I cut them. It is a time of reverence, remembrance, and hope. He asked, "What happens when they are all pink?"

I realized what he was asking and said, "I guess I will buy twelve more . . . twelve more with a pink one for every year she survives."

He smiled gleefully like I had forgotten something. "Why did you choose twelve roses to give her?"

I never told him the answer, but there is a certain day in October that I promised myself I would never forget.

George S.J. Anderson, RN
Dedicated to Lois A. Anderson, MT,
stage III breast cancer survivor,
diagnosed October 12, 1992, at age 39
Pennsylvania

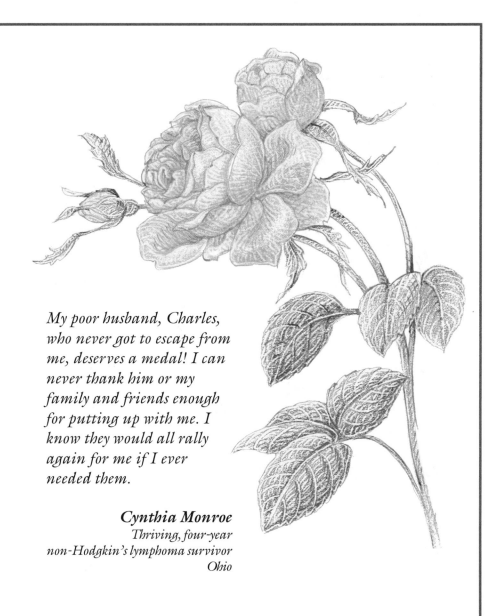

*My poor husband, Charles,
who never got to escape from
me, deserves a medal! I can
never thank him or my
family and friends enough
for putting up with me. I
know they would all rally
again for me if I ever
needed them.*

Cynthia Monroe
*Thriving, four-year
non-Hodgkin's lymphoma survivor
Ohio*

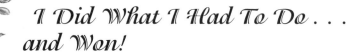

I Did What I Had To Do . . . and Won!

I detested vomiting and refused to do it. My oncologist was amused that I could talk myself out of it.

When the surgeon said "mastectomy," my mind rebelled. "No, I cannot have a mastectomy," I told myself. "I am getting married!"

However, reality quickly set in. I pushed my fear aside and decided to do what had to be done. I made a will. I cried! I packed for the hospital. I cried! By surgery time, I was calm, listening to an inner voice telling me that I was going to be all right. Perhaps the voice belonged to God or my guardian angel. I embraced this comfort. My daughter arrived just in time for kisses before surgery. When I awoke, she was there with my fiance. We were giddy with happiness because the cancer had spread to only two of my lymph nodes. We were so silly that night. When my fiance offered me my meal tray and asked "Would you like a pear?" I looked at my poor chest and replied, "I sure would!" Humor became our best medicine.

My daughter, who is an RN, stayed for the week and took care of my every need. Soon after, she had to return home, leaving my fiance and me to deal with the chemotherapy, injections, pills, bone scans, nausea, and hair loss. Nausea was not a problem for me. I detested vomiting and refused to do it. My oncologist was amused that I could talk myself out of it. My fiance would tease my thinning hair until light shone through. We laughed and cried as we counted each precious strand. The time came for me to show him my scar from surgery. I trembled with fear and shame but he kissed me tenderly as he looked at my chest, saying that he loved me even more because I was still with him. I knew then that the wedding was still on.

Our wedding day was beautiful. My oncologist gave me two weeks off my treatments. He was impressed with my fiance's strength and commitment. The minister placed chairs at the altar because I was too weak to stand through the ceremony.

After chemotherapy, radiation became my daily treatment. My doctors laughed when I told them I was designing my own bathing suit with huge ruffles at the bodice. During this time, I often shed tears, but many were tears of laughter as I adjusted to my new life. In the end, I found the challenge of recovery to be rewarding. I found courage, true love, and acceptance. My past struggles seemed minor, and life became more beautiful. I developed a new respect for myself. I have "graduated," as my oncologist would say, to live a fuller and more loving life. I did what I had to do and won! Twelve years later, I am still here!

Sally Ann Dolfi
Twelve-year breast cancer survivor
Florida

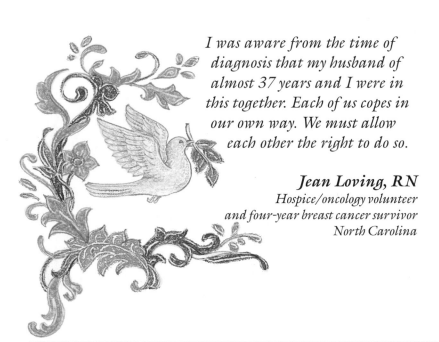

I was aware from the time of diagnosis that my husband of almost 37 years and I were in this together. Each of us copes in our own way. We must allow each other the right to do so.

Jean Loving, RN
Hospice/oncology volunteer
and four-year breast cancer survivor
North Carolina

Expressions of Love

How ironic that we must flirt with death to have a chance at life!

As I suppose most people are, I was totally unprepared for the diagnosis of inflammatory breast cancer that I received in August 1995. My doctor told me that my aggressive cancer had a poor prognosis, so I began chemotherapy treatment within days of confirming the diagnosis. A year of pain, illness, fear, and uncertainty followed, complete with chemotherapy, surgery, bone marrow transplant, and radiation. I was poked, prodded, poisoned, cut open, reassembled, and bombarded with invisible rays. How ironic that we must flirt with death to have a chance at life! Sounds like gray clouds indeed. Cancer is a harrowing experience. We must find ways to grow from the experience and give it meaning in our lives.

My prognosis now is looking much better. Two things that have seen me through this trial are my optimistic outlook on life and the wonderful, loving support I received from family, friends, and even people I do not know. I have been a caregiver in my personal and professional life. Cancer taught me how to graciously receive what others had to give me. The silver lining of my cancer storm has been to discover how many people truly love and care about me.

When I started chemotherapy, my friend Ellie began a tradition that she maintained during the following months. When I arrived home after my treatments, I would discover a package in my mailbox. Ellie would send a small gift wrapped in aluminum foil—a book, tape, lucky rock—with a reminder that "every chemotherapy treatment should have a silver lining." The silver lining was not the tangible gift, but Ellie herself. How she honored our friendship and found this way to be with me through my treatment was the best gift of all.

Ellie was just one of my silver linings. There also were Pam, who used her artistic magic to create a healing blanket and angels to watch over me; Nancy, who opened her heart and home so I could continue to work during my chemotherapy and avoid the usual two-hour commute; Katrina, with her nursing background, who volunteered to be my private night nurse after my surgery; and Mary, always practical, who sent two women to clean my house for a year and visited me every Friday night for what we came to call "Baldy's Happy Hour." Finally, there was Dan, my pilot friend, who called at least once a week from exotic (and not-so-exotic) places to let me know that his prayers were not diminished across the miles. These friends and so many others were among the silver linings of my cancer experience.

The most glowing silver lining has been the renewed closeness, depth, and mutual appreciation that has developed between me and those dearest to me: my husband, son, daughter, mother, and sister. Whatever happens in the future, I go forward knowing that I am loved. I have touched, and been touched by, many lives and loves.

Penny Cupp
Inflammatory breast cancer survivor
Georgia

Having cancer has continued to be a positive for me because of the character of everyone involved with cancer and its treatments. The commitment the staff made to "Camp Rising Spirits" is certainly one of the many ways that they go above and beyond the call of duty. They are very special people with arms for hugs, ears for listening, shoulders for tears, and hearts so big that they have room for all who come to them for comfort and reassurance. They know that there is no cure for the pain except LOVE, which they give abundantly. They are my silver linings that are the other side of cancer.

Nancy Dunnewold
Melanoma and breast cancer survivor
Pennsylvania

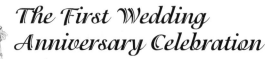

The First Wedding Anniversary Celebration

"Have you ever seen anyone more beautiful?"
Chad asked himself more than us.

I found the invitation written on a coffee-stained paper placemat. It read, "You are invited to celebrate our first wedding anniversary at 2 pm. No gifts. Just friends. Love, Chad and Mary Margaret."

He had the body of Fred Flintstone and dressed like "Nacho Man." She looked like a cross between Dorothy Hamill and Jackie Kennedy. He burped in public. She made television commercials. Chad was as healthy as a horse. Mary Margaret had breast cancer.

"There's no way I can go," I said to myself. I had to give a report, set up medications, and take care of patients. Besides, it was already two o'clock.

Suddenly, I heard the majestic organ chords of the "Wedding March" coming from Mary Margaret's room. "Well, maybe for just a minute," I decided. The other staff members must have thought the same thing. Everyone was already there.

As Chad narrated the wedding video, Mary Margaret sat on her hospital bed throne, clutching her withered lilac bouquet. Amid the tangled oxygen tubing, IV pumps, and suction equipment stood nurses, orderlies, and even a few patients vying for a peek at the screen.

"Have you ever seen anyone more beautiful?" Chad asked himself more than us.

With tears and grape juice, we toasted the bride and groom. Each one had a bite of stale wedding cake. And, love triumphed—for the moment.

When the celebration ended, Chad hung a sign on the doorknob that read, "Do not disturb—Honeymoon in progress."

Susan Pee Mixon, RN
Oncology nurse
Mississippi

Lullaby

Sometimes nursing care requires skills that we didn't learn in nursing school . . .

Jennifer was four years old when she was hospitalized for treatment of her leukemia. It was about 9 pm and I was winding up a long day at work as a pediatric oncology nurse specialist at Cleveland Clinic. I couldn't resist one final visit to her room to see how she was doing. I found her alone and crying. She looked so small as she was curled up in her huge hospital bed.

Tearfully, she told me that her mom had to go to work and she couldn't get to sleep. I was tired and really wanted to go home. Her staff nurse was busy with her other patients. I decided to read her a story to see if it would help her to fall asleep. After reading the story, she still couldn't relax enough to fall off to sleep. I climbed into her bed and curled up beside her tiny little body. I held her in my arms and began to sing to her as I stroked her hair. Within a short time, I could hear her rhythmic breathing. She was fast asleep.

Ann Birkmire, RN, MSN
Pediatric clinical nurse specialist
Massachusetts

I have come to admire my mother's resiliency. I am reminded afresh that one is forever changed by the cancer experience. With no current evidence of disease, my mom and I both share the survivor's role.

Joanne Hindle, RN, BSN, OCN®
Cancer survivor, oncology nurse,
and daughter of cancer survivor
Colorado

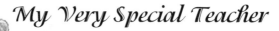

My Very Special Teacher

I will never, ever forget her. She is the best.

It was my first day in third grade.
I sat all tense and scared.
My teacher walked in and gave a smile.
I loved the way it made me feel inside.
My very special teacher.

When I was having bad days, she always made me happy.
She had lots of fun things for us to do.
She gave me many, many hugs throughout the day.
She was very laid back.
My very special teacher.

She told me some of her life stories.
I learned that she used to have cancer.
I asked her to teach me more about it.
She took me to a hospice center.
My very special teacher.

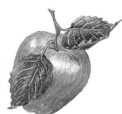

It was very sad to see the year come to an end.
I cried and cried.
I wished so hard that she could be my teacher again.
My wish came true!
My very special teacher.

I could not wait for fourth grade to begin.
The beginning of it was a blast.
Toward the middle of fourth grade, I became scared.
She was not acting like her cheerful self.
My very special teacher.

My mom talked to her to see what was happening.
I will never forget the day she called me to her desk.
She gave me a hug and looked into my eyes.
I knew what she was going to tell me.
My very special teacher.

She told me that her cancer had come back.
I froze, my eyes became teary, and I started to shake.
She gave me another hug that I can still feel.
I was worried for the rest of the year.
My very special teacher.

I was sad because she would never be my teacher again.
However, that summer I found out some good news.
Her cancer went away.
I was relieved.
My very special teacher.

As the years have gone by, she has had good times and bad.
I think of her often and say lots of prayers.
I will never, ever forget her. She is the best.
I love her very much!
My very special teacher, Mrs. Darlene Bierwagen.

Cammie Jackson
Seventh grader
Wyoming

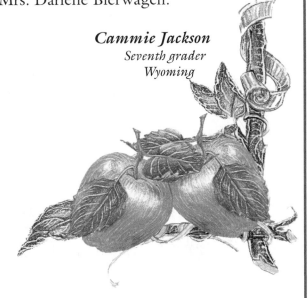

The Ambush

It is truly not possible for me to express to my family how much I appreci- ated that they interrupted their lives to be with me. And my friends? I have the best collection in the world!

It was a Saturday when the ambush occurred. I was taking a shower— a shower that lasted some four hours and 15 minutes—with the water running the entire time. What happened? I had a seizure. It must have been a whopper because I managed to push the shower door open, which allowed water to run throughout the house, thus flooding the bathroom, vanity area, bedroom, and sitting area!

Because I was expected to meet a colleague and never showed up, she pursued me via telephone and beeper. When there was no response, she called a friend who came to the house and discovered me. Apparently, I was quite a sight. I was sitting on the side of the bathtub, with wrinkled skin, dripping wet, and with a towel wrapped around me. My friend called 911, and an ambulance arrived to take me to the hospital. (I, of course, have no recollection of this.) The following is the story of my cancer and, frankly, not nearly as exciting as the shower escapade.

My friends clearly were as stunned as I was about this occurrence. After all, I was a 47-year-old female who had never taken a sick day in her life. I underwent the usual tests over the weekend and was advised that I had a brain tumor! I think this is when I really "woke up" follow- ing the seizure. I remember asking the neurologist, "Say that again? I have a what?" When he repeated "brain tumor," I asked if he could show it to me. Indeed, it was there, large as life, on the MRI film.

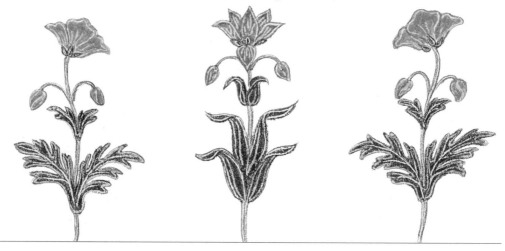

Two key activities followed in the next week: talking with my parents and three sisters and making arrangements to have this thing removed so I could get on with my life. Dealing with my parents was difficult. My oldest sister had a brain stem aneurysm just a year and one-half earlier. She survived the overwhelming surgery and rehabilitation and is now a fully functional individual. She returned to her responsibilities as an RN in record time. I had experienced the effect of her illness on my parents and knew how tough it was on the entire family. I am amazed at how protective I felt toward my folks! Although in their mid-70s, they are spry and energetic. We engineered a plan in which my sister would be at my folks' home so she could explain what I was saying.

I decided to have my craniotomy at Shands Hospital, University of Florida, rather than at my own healthcare facility. I think I decided on this hospital because of my sister's very successful surgery there and to escape my own facility where I was sure the staff would be a bit un-settled. One week after my diagnosis, I underwent the surgery without complications. I was discharged in three days and was able to return to work three weeks later. Why not? I was quite bored at home. Of course, I was very interested in the pathology of my tumor. After waiting 12 long days for my results, I learned that I had a low-medium grade tumor. I was reasonably pleased with this news because if one has to have a cancer, this one, I was told, was not an awful one to have. As expected, a neuropathologist at H. Lee Moffitt Cancer Center and a pathologist in Arizona reviewed my slides and blocks. After endlessly waiting, my physician confirmed that I had a low-grade tumor. The good news was that I required no chemotherapy! Needless to say, I was quite happy to hear this!

Five weeks after my craniotomy, I underwent seven weeks of radiation therapy. This was quite an experience. It was not the treatments them-selves that got to me; it was the almost sudden onset of fatigue. I decided that I would continue to work during my treatments. However, I probably worked too many hours. Plus, I had my treatments at the end of the long work day. I liked being the last appointment because I could go down after work, take off my scarf and earrings, and get "zapped." No big deal. The fatigue, on the other hand, *was* a big deal. I really thought I knew what fatigue was until I actually experienced it.

It is amazing how fatigue can control how much productive work one can do. I now feel better able to talk with patients about fatigue and manage ways to deal with it.

I definitely believe that I have received so much during this experience. Because I am not accustomed to receiving, I learned that I needed to accept the abundance of cards, flowers, plants, and food from so many people. I could have stocked a card and a flower shop with the gifts I received! I did not have to cook for weeks! It is not possible for me to express to my family how much I appreciated that they interrupted their lives to be with me. I also have found that I have the best collection of friends in the world. No joke! As I continue to follow the defined course with frequent MRIs, I often reflect on the puzzlement of that ambush followed by my successful surgery and therapy. I do know that the good Lord is not ready for me just yet. He has bigger plans for me down here!

Linda R. Campbell, RN, MS
Nurse administrator and brain tumor survivor
Florida

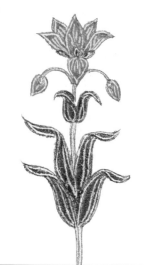

Revealing raw emotion and baring your soul . . . unending devotion and unconsciously becoming numb to endure the pain . . . rising above the fear . . . loving more than you thought humanly possible and not knowing if it will ever be enough . . . this is dealing with cancer. You love so hard it hurts. You listen more intently than you imagined possible. These are the feelings worth sharing . . . with my best friend . . . my sister . . . my soul mate.

Nancy S. Hardy-Jennings
Sister of breast cancer survivor
Iowa

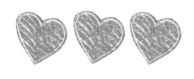

Another Day Together

Life is so limited regardless of cancer. Learn to enjoy it.

During my first year of college in 1976, I met a gentleman with whom I shared many of the same classes. Our eyes met. We eventually started studying together and sharing conversations. I soon learned that he was undergoing treatment for Hodgkin's disease, so I accompanied him on many of his hospital visits. During the trips for treatments and our time spent studying together for classes, we bonded. We never shared a dull or unsatisfying moment, regardless of the circumstances. We enjoyed life to the fullest! However, he graduated before me and left the state in search of job opportunities.

Throughout the years, we continued to correspond. His cancer returned in 1986. Consequently, more treatments followed. Although we lived in different states and maintained different life-styles, our close bond never diminished. In 1988, we married, and in 1992, he underwent a bone marrow transplant. We both felt optimistic about the "adventure" of the transplant because each new adventure meant another day spent together. Life is so limited regardless of cancer. One must learn to enjoy it.

Family and friends love to come to our home; we always have an abundance of fun, food, music, conversation, and warmth. For whatever reason or cause, my family has been blessed. My husband still has his health, and we have another day together.

Renne Denise Johansen
Wife and companion to a man
with Hodgkin's disease
Nebraska

The Most Beautiful Woman
in the World

*"There is nothing that could make me stop loving you.
You are the love of my life!"*

In March 1966, I had just celebrated my 36th birthday. While I was bathing, I found a small lump about the size of a marble on the outside of my left breast. I was not greatly alarmed. I had my yearly checkup in January and was accustomed to finding fibrocystic lumps. However, my husband insisted that I see a physician immediately. Two weeks later, on March 31, 1966, I was on the operating table, hopefully just to have a biopsy. However, I was told that if the lump was malignant, a radical mastectomy would be performed immediately. I was sure I would be home the following day to celebrate my daughter's sixth birthday.

I awoke at 6 o'clock that evening to learn I had been on the operating table for five-and-one-half hours. My left breast, lymph glands, and part of my chest muscle were gone. The tumor was malignant! I immediately made up my mind that I would do whatever it would take to live. I could not die when I had two young children to care for. I had to live to see them as adults.

It was one full year before I could raise my left arm. I continued to have biopsies of my right breast. In 1968, I had another lump removed that was diagnosed as an enlarged lymph node. I decided that I could not go through the anxiety of having biopsies every six months, so I had a simple mastectomy of my right breast.

Perhaps my most cherished memory is when I came home from the hospital for the very first time. I could hardly look at my chest. I could not stand the weight of my blouse against my skin, and a bra was totally out of the question, so my disfigurement was very obvious. I felt that no one could ever look at me again without a shudder. My husband kissed me, helped me change, and said, "There is nothing that could ever make me stop loving you. You are the love of my life and the most beautiful woman in the world to me!" I cried for the very first time.

I was sure this would be my last bout with this disease. I spent almost 20 years cancer-free—if anyone who has ever had cancer can truly feel free of cancer. However, in August 1986, I found another lump in my right thigh that turned out to be a totally new cancer. This was a tumor of the skin and connecting tissue and was not related to my breast cancer. Once again, the lump was removed with a wide excision.

I am now 65 years old and soon will celebrate my 45th wedding anniversary with the same wonderful man. I have seen my son's marriage and the birth of my two granddaughters. I cared for my mother until her death. I visit my daughter regularly. I am free of cancer and living every day with a great respect for the gift of a healthy body. I do aqua aerobics three times a week, babysit my grandchildren whenever I can, fish with my husband, sew, write, and dream. Most of all, I thank God for the blessing of life as I awaken to each new day. Sometimes I think of the physicians who saved my life and ask God to save a special place in heaven for them.

Georgina K. Frei
Grandmother, mother, wife, and
30-year breast cancer survivor
California

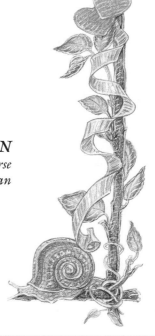

EACH DAY BLOSSOMS
into fullness
amid love's light
that shines from within
and opens outward
as tenderly as a rose.

Christine Umscheid, RN
Breast cancer survivor and oncology nurse
Michigan

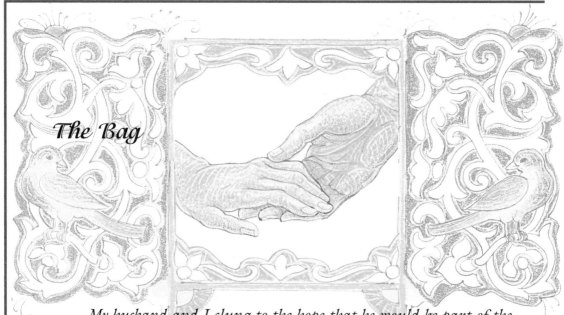

The Bag

My husband and I clung to the hope that he would be part of the 30% of survivors of this disease; after all, that 30% had to hold someone. Why not him?

My husband was diagnosed with an advanced stage of colorectal cancer three years ago. The cancer had metastasized to his liver. After surgery, he was discharged with an ileostomy. He experienced the normal surgical routine in the hospital and tried to comply with the instructions for diet, ambulation, and ostomy care. He made follow-up appointments with the surgeon and the medical and radiation oncologists. My husband and I clung to the hope that he would be part of the 30% of survivors of this disease; after all, that 30% had to hold *someone*. Why not him? At the time of his diagnosis, we had six children and four grandchildren, all of whom lived out of state, except our youngest daughter who was in college two-and-one-half hours away. Sounds like a typical family, right?

Did I neglect to mention that my husband is a general practitioner/ family practice physician with a speciality in sports medicine who also played professional football for seven years? Did I mention that I am an oncology clinical nurse specialist at a regional cancer center? One of our daughters also is an oncology nurse in Atlanta, GA. Our family is half healthcare professionals and half sports professionals.

My husband and I were always sensitive to our patients' feelings and knew how stressful a cancer diagnosis can be. Yet, I truly cannot express the stinging pain in my heart that this would happen to such a kind and generous husband, father, and small-town physician, even though I see it every day at work. I honestly can say (and my coworkers will agree) that I absolutely could not speak to anyone about his cancer for six weeks because I would burst into tears. We both desperately wanted to overcome this. We had the knowledge and expertise to do it. The biggest challenge, believe it or not, was "the bag!" Not the chemotherapy or radiation treatments, but "the bag."

I should have realized that someone who was always physically active and athletic would struggle with his body image. How he *hated* "the bag." As a nurse, I should have known better. In the past, I had enough knowledge of ostomies to get by, but as many staff nurses do, I always called the enterostomal specialist when I encountered problems. After all, she was the expert, and I had so many other tasks to complete.

Out of this experience, my husband and I discovered our silver lining. It was a few days before Christmas, and we were having accident after accident with the ostomy bags. They were leaking and falling off. He was developing sores everywhere. We both were frustrated, crying, and angry. I could not figure out what in the world we were doing wrong. Finally, I called the supplier, thinking I had received a shipment of faulty equipment. He suggested that I pick up a new supply before the holiday weekend—free of charge.

When I returned home and tried the new bags, we experienced the very same problems as before. Over the next 24 hours, we had even more accidents. I was washing constantly and cleaning everything in sight because our family was coming home for the holidays, and at this point, neither one of us wanted to deal with visitors, much less children who were grieving over these circumstances.

Finally, I looked through my purse and found the name of the enterostomal therapist with whom I had worked at a previous hospital. I called her in tears, sobbing that I did not know what I was doing wrong and nothing seemed to be working. I felt stupid and helpless, like I was not a good caregiver at all! After describing my problems to her, she said that my husband's stoma probably had shrunk and the hole for the ostomy bag was too big. Of course, that's why the bag would not stay on and sores were developing.

Her solution was to recut the opening of the bag and refit it to the stoma, not to use adhesive cream (it stings), and only use powder and the heat from my husband's body and my hand to hold the bag in place for a good three to five minutes. In desperation, I decided to give this a try, but I had such a headache from crying and my nose and eyes were so swollen that I could hardly concentrate.

I discovered that the process was much nicer if we lay together in bed and cuddled under the covers for a few minutes to make sure the seal held tight. It worked! In fact, that bag stayed on for two whole days after Christmas. We were so pleased that when the time came to change the bag, we feared we would not have the same success. But we went through the "cuddle routine" again. We found a new private time just for us.

When we had to change the bag, our cuddling became routine, day or night. It became a time of togetherness. I assured my husband that I still loved to be close to him physically. This made him realize that no bag could come between us. I did not realize until later that our cuddle time made my husband's ileostomy experience easier. It brought us together both physically and emotionally. We cried, we prayed, and we healed during this time.

Since that time, my husband was fortunate to have his ileostomy reversed. However, without the experience of "that bag," we never would have learned that our cuddle time was so precious. We often look back on those trying days and reflect on what he considered to be such a physically demeaning time for him. As a spouse, I learned the importance of reassuring my husband that a physical change could never alter our intimacy.

Out of the dark clouds often comes a silver lining that brings couples even closer together. I tell my patients every day not to forget the importance of touch. It is the best therapy possible.

Kathy Adamle, RN, MSN, AOCN
Wife of husband with colon cancer
Ohio

Let Us Think of Hands

I have lived five years since I was first treated for breast cancer. It was a struggle with three surgeries, chemotherapy, and radiation treatments. I have lived to see my grandson born and watch him grow. I have so much love and support from family, friends, and medical people. I enjoy life and learned that we all help each other grow and heal. My experience with cancer inspired this poem.

Let us think of Hands.
Hands are for Touching,
Hands are for Healing,
We can all learn how.
Hands work, they play, make music, and art.
Hands Dance.
They mend nets, point telescopes, make lace, operate.
Hands know pain, a prick, a burn, a break, rheumatism.
But Hands know Healing.
Acknowledge the pain, hold it, and let it go.
Get to know your own hands,
Greet them each morning, let them give thanks,
And joy, and comfort.
Hands focus your thoughts.
They guide your prayers, in many positions.
Hands send messages to people earthwide.
Letters, telephones, computers—all need hands.
Next time you shake hands,
Hold on a little longer, give love, give healing.
Don't be afraid, they are your hands—gentle
And firm, never hitting in anger.
Hands do heal.
May the Divine Hold you by the Hand.

Ingrid M. Wing
Five-year breast cancer survivor
Ohio

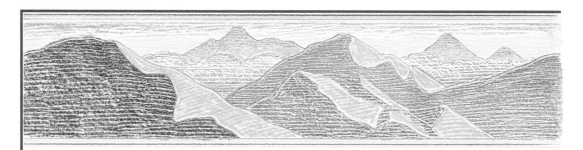

A Survivor's Story

The prayers took wings, and people reached out to our family in love.

The naked figure staring back at me from the bathroom mirror was an image so foreign that I struggled to make myself believe that it was really me. The loss of my silky brown hair exposed a bony, bare scalp. Dark eyes stared out of a thin face lacking brows and lashes—giving me the look of a space alien. Beneath my protruding collarbone sprouted a double-lumen catheter, saving me from constant needles and providing access for my chemotherapy, antibiotics, blood, platelets, antinausea drugs, and whatever else I needed to be kept alive. I cleaned the catheter meticulously and flushed it with heparin daily to keep it from clogging or developing an infection. It dumped right into my heart, which pumped the toxic, lifesaving chemotherapy throughout my body. Where my large breasts had once hung were two diagonal scars. My formerly rounded belly and hips vanished, as did my pubic hair. My legs looked like sticks. Nausea replaced my appetite.

I lived in outpatient housing near Stanford Medical Center in California for three months. I received the highest doses of chemotherapy given, followed by three bone marrow transplants in an experimental stem cell rescue protocol. I felt fortunate to be accepted into such a program. At 42 years of age, I had been diagnosed with stage IV breast cancer that had metastasized to my lymph nodes and bone marrow. I missed my husband of 18 years, Bill, and our beautiful 14-year-old twin sons, Nick and Peter, who were 200 miles away. Each day I prayed for God to give me the strength to survive the massive hits of chemotherapy and the multitude of side effects.

"There is always a miracle, Barbara," my surgeon had said to me before I entered treatment. That is what my church, friends, and family were praying for. The prayers took wings, and people reached

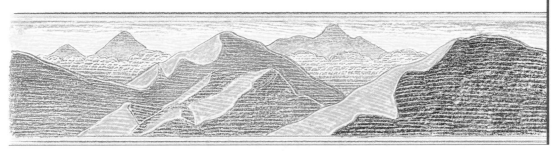

out to our family in love. As a teacher, I received tremendous support from my entire school district. The staff used their personal days to take care of me at the hospital while my husband stayed home to run the business and care for our sons. Teachers and other friends came for three days at a time. They took me to the hospital and cared for me in my weakness. They were my cheerleaders. Bill, Nick, and Peter visited me every weekend. Friends at home provided months of meals for our family.

After my third transplant, I had a 104° fever for eight days. With my body packed in ice, I fought vomiting, diarrhea, and a lung inflammation. I felt that I was in the "valley of the shadow of death" and prayed the words of Psalm 23 in my hospital bed. Miraculously, I survived that dark time and went home 10 days later. Two years later, my tests prove that I am still cancer-free. Yes, Virginia, God still does make miracles.

Barbara C. Spangler
Mother with stage IV breast cancer and
bone marrow transplant survivor
California

Finding Love and a Chance to Help Others

"So many wonderful things have come from my bout with leukemia that I almost look upon it as a blessing. God certainly has seen to it that my suffering did not go without its rewards!"

Karen Quigley and her husband, Matthew, conducted their courtship on the bone marrow transplant unit at George Washington University Hospital in Washington, DC. The couple met through Matthew's sister, an oncology nurse who cared for Karen during her first bout with leukemia in 1993.

"My sister-in-law, Jane, was a large part of my discovering the silver lining in my cancer. She was always kidding about wanting me to meet her brother in Baton Rouge," Karen said. "After I got out, we came here on a trip, and I met him. He is a chemical engineer. It was love at first sight. I didn't tell him I had cancer until my relapse in August of 1994. At that point, a bone marrow transplant was recommended. He was great. He told me he had waited 26 years for the right woman; he could wait a little longer. He flew up to see me every other weekend, and we were engaged while I was still in the hospital."

Following a 75-day recuperation stay on the unit, Karen married Matthew and moved to Louisiana. She now works part-time for Cancer Services of Baton Rouge as the only cancer survivor on staff. She also is facilitating a new bone marrow transplant support group in her town.

"I am excited to be working with the support group. I was part of a group in Washington, DC, and it meant a lot to me, both in terms of moral support and exchange of information," said Quigley.

Half a dozen patients who have undergone bone marrow transplants attended the first few meetings. Quigley said the group talked about holding monthly meetings, acting as a resource for new patients, and possibly sponsoring a bone marrow drive in the future. All of the attendees at the first meetings underwent transplants elsewhere.

Quigley feels good now. She is off all medication and returns for check ups every eight months. She enjoys working again, and she and her husband are buying a house. "Baton Rouge is my home now," she said. "The people I work with are like my family. I feel blessed. A lot of people helped me get where I am today, and if I can help someone else, then I would like that. I do not have a social work degree, but I have been there. So many wonderful things have come from my bout with leukemia that I almost look upon it as a blessing. My family and I firmly believe that God has a reason behind everything that occurs in life. God certainly has seen to it that my suffering did not go without its rewards!"

From "Woman Facilitating Local Support Group,"
by Laurie Smith Anderson. Reprinted from the August 5, 1996 issue
by permission of The Advocate, Baton Rouge, LA.

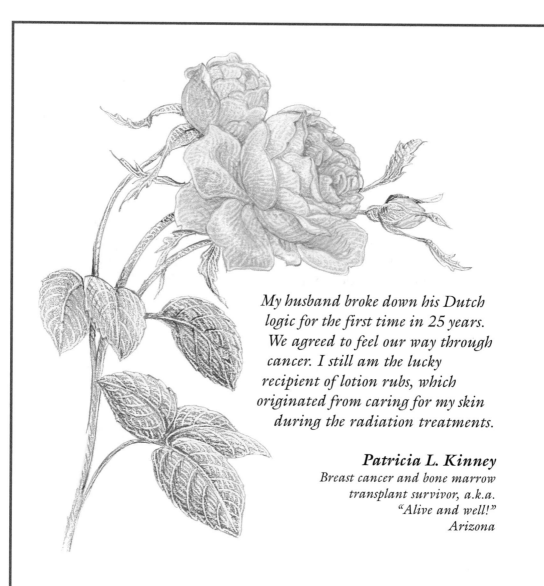

My husband broke down his Dutch
logic for the first time in 25 years.
We agreed to feel our way through
cancer. I still am the lucky
recipient of lotion rubs, which
originated from caring for my skin
during the radiation treatments.

Patricia L. Kinney
Breast cancer and bone marrow
transplant survivor, a.k.a.
"Alive and well!"
Arizona

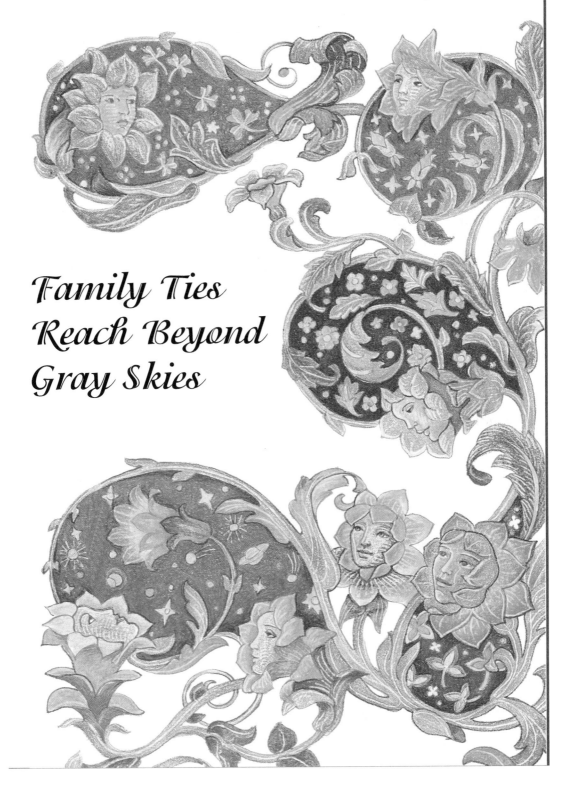

Chapter 3

Family Ties Reach Beyond Gray Skies

Show Me the Good in This Crappy Day

In that single moment, God showed me "the purpose"
of that crappy day, and I gave thanks for it!

Mother's Day 1994 is a day I will remember always. It wasn't a traditional Mother's Day with a Hallmark card, flowers, and lunch out at McDonald's. It was a sobering, transforming day—a day filled with mixed and powerful emotions and experiences.

My daughter, Lisa, was not quite 15 that Mother's Day, and my son, Jim, had just turned 13 a few weeks earlier. I had two teenagers, both of whom were suffering from what I called hormone poisoning. To complicate my life even more, I was four months into chemotherapy for treatment of Hodgkin's disease. Needless to say, it was a pretty rough period. We were all, in our own way, facing the most challenging and frightening journey of our lives.

Once I "got out of my head and into my heart," after I moved beyond intellectualizing my situation and permitted myself to feel what I was experiencing, I found a place of courage, hope, and understanding. My children had a much harder time coping and feeling what they were going through. That Mother's Day, however, was a turning point for at least one of my children.

As long as I live, I'll never forget how sick and drained I felt that day. I had just finished a round of chemotherapy, and my blood count was very low. My antiemetics weren't working, and I had a terrible head and chest cold. Every part of my body ached. All I wanted to do was cry, but I didn't have the energy. I was exhausted! I did, however, manage to get heavily into my "pity-party" and the "poor me's." I recall asking—actually, more like demanding—"God, show me the good in this crappy day. What is its purpose?" I couldn't wait for the day to be over.

Lisa and Jim spent the day with their dad, so when they came home that evening, they presented me with my Mother's Day gift. I really wasn't in the spirit of celebration, but I just couldn't disappoint them. They gave me an answering machine. Jim seemed so proud of their choice. He said, "Now you don't have to get up and answer the phone when you don't feel good, Mom. Happy Mother's Day."

I'd no sooner thanked them when a wave of nausea hit me and I threw up. With that, the mood changed. The party was over. Lisa flew off to her room and closed the door. Her room was her sanctuary; her safety zone; the place where she tried to escape from her fears, her sadness, her anger; the space where cancer was not allowed. How I grew to hate the sound of her closing that door! She would turn on her music in hopes of silencing life on the outside. My daughter had distanced herself from me and especially from her feelings since the very beginning of this "cancer thing." Even good-bye hugs and good-night kisses stopped. She never cried—at least not in front of me. For the first time in her life, I could not help or comfort her. Lisa's peace would come later.

After Lisa left the room, Jim became very quiet, which was quite unlike him. He handled his fears in a much different way. He was a one-man circus, a clown, a comedian. He'd try anything to make me laugh and help time pass more quickly for the both of us. We'd play cards, watch movies, and take short walks (mostly for ice cream).

Once Jim felt it was "safe," he sat down next to me on the couch, rested his arm around my shoulders, and squeezed tightly. Then, in almost a whisper, he asked, "Are you okay, Mom?" I said, "Yes. You don't have to stay." But he did.

My son looked scared. I could see worry and sadness in his eyes—eyes that couldn't look into mine. They were fixed in a forward, distant stare and blinking rapidly in an attempt to fight back his tears (he was, you know, at an age where only wussies cry). His breathing was deep and mechanical, and I could feel his body quiver with each breath. Every muscle in his being was tense. I could feel his fear, his confusion, his pain. I then rested my head on top of his and told him, "I love you, and I . . . we will all make it through this." With that, I watched his tears roll down his cheeks. He finally allowed himself to cry . . . for me and, most importantly, for himself. He let go.

Almost immediately, I could feel the tension in his body melt away, and I held him and rocked him like I did when he was little and afraid. In that single moment, God showed me "the purpose" of that crappy day, and I gave thanks for it!

Susan Hoag
Two-year lymphoma survivor
Ohio

Hearts

*Every day with my family feels like Mother's Day
and Valentine's Day all rolled into one.*

They were everywhere: on mirrors, pillows, and closed doors. You'd think it was coming—Mother's Day, that is. But it wasn't Mother's Day or even Valentine's Day. It was just Tuesday. And they—the hearts—all started appearing because I had cancer.

My children were not yet two, four, and six years old when I was diagnosed with lymphoma. The chemotherapy that followed sent my blood counts plummeting, making it unwise for me to be around my runny-nosed little ones. My husband, Ted, suggested they make hearts—paper hearts—for me so I could feel their love when I was sick in bed or away in the hospital. Rebecca's elaborate hearts with misspelled messages, Jessica's wordless hearts, and William's misshapen hearts sent perfect love my way. As the months of treatment turned into years, I wrote a book, *Becky and the Worry Cup,* to help my children (and others, too) find ways to combat the loneliness and sense of helplessness that can accompany a parent's cancer. In it, I included how Becky drew hearts.

Two years ago, during one of my remissions, I read the latest draft to William, now a vivacious six-year-old who had heard none of the earlier versions and remembered little of the actual events surrounding my chemotherapy. Ironically, a few weeks later a routine checkup revealed progressive disease for which another course of chemotherapy was advised. When I informed my children, William said nothing. That night, after I had put him to bed, I began my daily exercise workout. William silently crept into my room with an armful of new drawings. He laid them out on my bed, leaving a big pink paper heart on my pillow. When I caught sight of him, he explained, with a smile, "I'm practicing for when your counts are low."

The treatments worked well—I am once again in remission. But the fatigue has been slower to disappear than the cancer, and I still need a nap every afternoon. A few weeks back, as I closed my eyes for my daily rest, I heard a rustling noise. Curious, I got up to check and found a note in Jessica's handwriting taped to my door: "Everyone Keep Out! (except Dad)." No signature at the bottom—just a little heart. Yesterday, a cardboard heart was slipped under my door as I was writing on my computer. It read, "I love you, Mom. William." Hearts have blossomed in our home. Every day with my family feels like Mother's Day and Valentine's Day all rolled into one.

Wendy S. Harpham, MD
Author of After Cancer, Diagnosis Cancer, When a Parent Has Cancer, *and* Becky and the Worry Cup
Texas

I guess in a way, I was transported back to my childhood. A time when life was simpler and was to be enjoyed to the fullest. I now am appreciative of a beautiful sunrise and the little cardinal that sings outside my office window. I find friendships very precious, and they should always be treasured. I have learned to take the time I need for myself, whether it's to take a hot bath, read a good book, or just catnap on the couch.

Renee Behrens
Breast cancer survivor
Illinois

All the Love Poured Out on Me Has Healed Me

"Have faith in God and focus on the things you love."—Caterina
When filled with love, there is just no room in our hearts for fear,
guilt, anger, and anxiety.—Maria, her daughter

Caterina is a quiet, unassuming, 85-year-old woman. She was born in Europe and moved to the United States with our family late in her life. Hardships and loss are familiar to her, having experienced wars, displacement, and uncertainties most of her life. Caterina is my mother and the one I always turned to when I was troubled. The calm in her eyes and her soft, soothing words always reassure me. Caterina's approach to every problem was always the same: "Have faith in God and focus on the things you love." For her, this meant her family.

With her advancing age, Caterina's challenges have taken the form of illness. A heart attack nearly ended her life a few years ago. Then colon cancer challenged her with another surgery. The doctors were honest with us. They told us that she might not make it through another year. With her usual serenity, her concern was to spare us from worrying, reassuring us that if death must come, she was well-prepared and unafraid.

My brother and sisters and I were not so well-prepared. It hurt to think of what was ahead for our mother. The common thoughts associated with cancer—visions of suffering, gradual wasting, and the unavoidable loss—were things that none of us was able to accept. We all experienced sadness. We were tired, and we disagreed about the course of action to take for her care. Privately, we worried about the toll Mom's disease and treatment would take on our families and jobs. Yet, each time we saw Caterina, she had a smile for us. Pure joy was in her eyes as she beheld each one of us. All of my worries seemed to dissipate when I was with her, just as they did when I was a small child. The love that radiated from her filled me with peace and spilled over into my conversations with my brother and sisters. Soon, we began to work together, each doing whatever we could without making demands on one another. Things began to fall into place. I even looked forward to my share of driving Caterina to her doctor's appointments because the time we spent together in the waiting rooms became opportunities to talk about many things we just never seemed to have time to talk about before.

Today, the doctors are amazed at how well Caterina has recovered. Two years have passed, and she is still cancer-free and has returned to her normal activities. "It seems like a miracle," my sister said as we shared the good news. Our mother just smiled and said, "I was ready to die, but I could not go yet. All the love that you poured on me has healed me." I think the healing has not been for her alone; each one of us also has been healed—of fear, guilt, anger, and anxiety. There is just no room for those feelings in the hearts that Caterina helped to fill with love.

Maria Gamiere
Daughter of Caterina, a colon cancer survivor
Ohio

After many prayers, surgery, chemotherapy, and radiation, today, one year later, I'm sitting on top of a mountain with the leaves just starting to change. My husband and four-year-old son are exploring the hillside. It's a beautiful day! I thank God for this day and every second I have with my family.

Brenda Wilson
Wife, mother, and cancer survivor
Tennessee

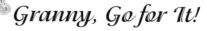

Granny, Go for It!

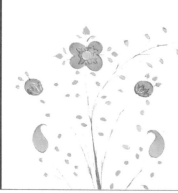

"Everybody knows you have cancer and are taking chemo. Who cares about hair!"

Two summers ago, I joined my children and grandchildren at the beach. The first day, they wanted me to play in the ocean with them. I had just started chemotherapy, so I had little hair. I asked my kids if this was embarrassing to them because I would need to take off my hat to swim. My 12-year-old grandson chimed in, "Oh, gee, Granny—everybody knows you have cancer and are taking chemo. Who cares about hair?" My stay in the ocean was as short as the waves were rough. When I started out, I asked the 12-year-old, "Want to catch a wave with me?" He nodded yes, so we body-surfed to the beach. When I came out of the surf, he raised his fist in the air and yelled, "All right, Granny, go for it!" Perfect advice, and I'm going to continue to do just that.

Myrtle Williams
*Wife, mother, grandmother, and
three-year ovarian cancer survivor
Georgia*

*I thank God for allowing me the
opportunity to see my grandchildren
grow up. Each day that I spend with
them is a special blessing.*

(Helen) Paulette Pyles
*Young grandmother and
30-month breast cancer survivor
Ohio*

Lucky to Have Her

She never gives up or loses hope.

The person I admire very much is my mother. She has done so much for both my family and me. Also, she has been a great role model and is a very inspiring person. One of her greatest qualities is her sense of humor and love for people. One of the most important things she has done for me is raising me in church and teaching me how to be nice and respectful to others. I really admire my mother for how she never gives up or loses hope. I also admire the way she kept her faith in God while she had cancer. She never thought for one second that He wasn't going to be there with her. She always knew that she would get better. Because of her faith, she has made a rapid recovery from cancer.

My mother is one of those women who will do almost anything for anybody. She is very sweet, caring, and loving toward others, and that has made her the great person that she is. In conclusion, I love my mother very much, and I am lucky to have her.

Bret Huskey
Age 14, son of Rita Huskey, four-and-one-half-year survivor of breast cancer
Tennessee

To cope with her illness, Mary concocted a plan to make a game of chemotherapy. When she went bald, she covered her head with aluminum foil and pretended with her children that she was really Materamus from the Planet Chemo. Laughing at the Chemo Creature Monster became the best way to allay their fears.

Morry Edwards, PhD
Doctor of Mary, a patient with lymphoma
Michigan

Gifts That I May Never Have Found

*My life has never been the same since
I was diagnosed with cancer.
I have made so many new discoveries.*

While on vacation in Ohio's Amish country in the summer of 1994, I noticed a pain below my belt line. After many tests and a biopsy, I was diagnosed as having large cell lymphoma. I found myself asking, "Why? Why would this happen to me? I went to church and tried to be a good person. I worked very hard. Why me?" I had to build two homes from the bottom up in addition to working my full-time job. My wife, children, and I are close. However, even though my wife and I are from large families, we never knew them because of family strife that occurred before we were old enough to be a part of it. The thought hit me: If I died, none of my cousins and other family members would have any memories me.

As a result of my illness, we changed the way our families interacted. Now we meet (about 50 of us in all) every other month at someone's home or a park for a day of getting to know each other. We are making happy memories now and sharing the many aspects of our lives that we never shared before.

I traveled many valleys on my journey to recovery from cancer. I never stayed in the low valleys for long. I had many people all over the country praying for me, and my new grandchild gave me the will to keep going. As people sent me cards, I lined them up along a large mirror. This did two things: It kept me from seeing my bald head and pale skin, and it also gave me a tremendous lift to see all the people who cared about me and were praying for me. A relative of one of my customers let my wife and family use their home while I was in the hospital. My sisters would cook meals and freeze them so that we did not have to worry about meals when we finally returned home from the hospital. My life has never been the same since I was diagnosed with cancer. I have made so many new discoveries in my life.

My outlook on life is so different now. I am more sensitive to all the love around me. I take time to enjoy the simple things in life. I am a part of my family; they know me, and I know them. Cancer is a devastating disease, but it has given me many gifts that I may never have found.

Doug Jones
Husband, father, and lymphoma survivor
Michigan

The hardest thing for us to face was when I heard the doctor say the word cancer. *We've also realized how much we care about and need each other—more than we possibly could have imagined. I know one thing— with everything that has happened to us, our relationship as a family has never been stronger. We keep growing stronger every day.*

Linda Allard
Part of a family fighting together
California

The Cancer Changed Him

Sam explained how the cancer had changed him—he was a "people person" now and wanted to spend time with Jay. Sam said he could not afford to lose his son again—not now.

I met Jay while he was working in the radiology department of our cancer hospital. We were at lunch one day when Jay told me that his father had prostate cancer and was terminal. As Jay spoke of his father, he repeated, "I don't care what happens to him. It's his own fault because he ignored the symptoms." Jay went on to explain how his relationship with his father was poor, even nonexistent at times. They would not speak for weeks at a time.

Fate intervened, and within one month of our conversation, Sam (Jay's father) was admitted to the hospital for pain control and to rule out sepsis. On the third day of Sam's hospitalization, his pain was under control. With some pushing from his mom, Jay went to see his father. Jay asked me to come into the room with him. As Sam's nurse, I did so, just in case Sam became agitated or needed emotional support. I remember the room being dark and Jay walking cautiously over to the side of the bed. I remained by the door. The two men started speaking slowly, and both were searching for things to say. Then, Sam asked Jay to sit down. Jay later told me that he expected a lecture. Instead, Sam told his son he loved him and he was proud of him. Jay was quiet for a moment and then responded with, "I love you too, Dad." At this point, I stepped out of the room, giving them some much-needed time alone. When I checked on them later, both men had been crying. The conversation appeared a little easier. Sam explained how the cancer had changed him—he was a "people person" now and wanted to spend time with Jay. Sam said he could not afford to lose his son again—not now.

All of Jay's and Sam's differences have not been, and will not be, resolved. They have not become the best of friends. According to Jay, it took Sam's cancer diagnosis to recognize what was important in life: not the money, not the cars, not the boats, but rather his family and making the time left together quality time.

Elizabeth Bertelli-Whidden, RN, BSN
Bone marrow transplant and
neuro-oncology nurse
Florida

I learned to make the most of everything—both the good and the bad. I appreciate more than ever all the simple things that we normally take for granted. My family became more important than ever to me. My motto is "Enjoy everything while we can—it's later than we think."

Tina Kapsanis
Bilateral breast cancer survivor
Florida

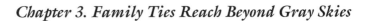

A Miracle in the Shadows

*Amidst the shadows of the dark cloud
that cancer brought to me,
a miracle happened.*

Sometimes, no matter how strong our faith, we question what we believe. When I was stricken with non-Hodgkin's lymphoma at age 27, I was angry at God. I had spent my entire adult life working to stay physically fit and healthy. I prided myself on being a friendly, outgoing individual. So, why did this happen to me? How can bad things happen to good people? Well, only God can truly answer these questions . . . and perhaps when things like cancer happen, He doesn't have anything to do with it at all. I can tell you that in my life, amidst the shadows of the dark cloud that cancer brought to me, a miracle happened. I would like to cast the shadow aside and focus on that miracle.

Sometime in the late summer of 1991 my wife, Lara, and I made a split-second decision to have a child. I know how that sounds, but keep in mind that this is where the miracle begins. Shortly thereafter, we decided that perhaps we had been hasty and were not ready for children, so we would be more careful. It was not long after that singular incident that Lara discovered that she was pregnant! Well, earlier sentiments aside, we could not have been happier. In November of 1991, my job carried me to Cambodia where I was to spend 60 days preparing for the opening of the new American Embassy. It was an exciting job. Cambodia was a dismal place, though, just crawling back from years of strife under the Khmer Rouge. The health conditions were terrible. When I returned home in January, I was not feeling quite up to par. I couldn't lay my finger on it, but I was tired almost all of the time.

A few months later, while lifting weights, I experienced pain along my rib cage. While showering, I found a small, peanut-sized lump on my chest, and it was very painful. My doctor initially diagnosed it as an inflamed tendon from a muscle pull. When a second lump appeared on my neck, we began to get concerned. Following a biopsy of the second lump, my worst fears were confirmed. I had a high-grade non-Hodgkin's lymphoma. I was to undergo chemotherapy immediately.

How could this be happening to me? What would I tell my wife? We had been praying that this would wind up being nothing serious. At the very worst, we thought maybe I had come down with some strange tropical disease. But cancer—we tried not to even think about it. Funny how that one word can make your whole world come crashing down. Everything you believe in comes into question.

In consultations with my oncologist, he suggested that if I wanted children, I should consider making deposits in the bank of life (euphemistically speaking). I told him that my wife was expecting, and if one child was all we were destined to have, then so be it! It wasn't until later that evening that Lara and I discovered just how miraculous this pregnancy was. When we thought about how close we had come to the real danger of not being able to have children, it made that split-second decision that we had made the previous summer seem more like divine intervention! So, I entered my chemotherapy with the relief that I would be the father of at least one child.

Our son, Christian, was born June 4, 1992. He is an amazing four-year-old with a bright future ahead of him. His sister, Lindsay, our second miracle, is a beautiful one-year-old with wonder in her eyes. I firmly believe that God does not pull all of the strings—
just the ones that count.

Darren G. Riggs
Non-Hodgkin's lymphoma survivor
U.S. State Department, Finland

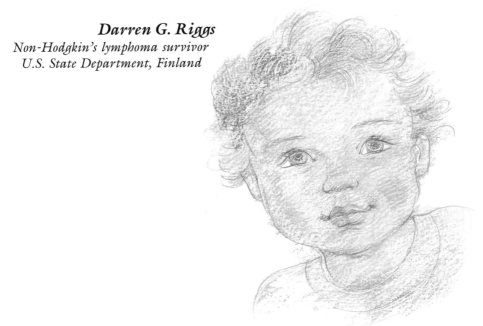

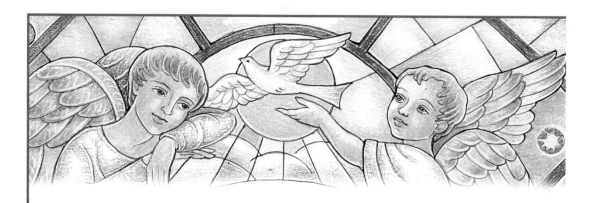

A Reason to Go On

From that moment, I began to gain strength and
believed there was some reason for me to go on.

More than four years ago, blood in my stool sent me to the doctor in Naples, FL. He gave me tests and medicine, but my wife and I decided to move back to our home in Minnesota for follow-up treatment.

One day, with time on my hands, I drove to the hospital for a prescription refill. While waiting for my pills, the doctor suggested I get a physical. Soon, I heard my name over the PA system instructing me to report to the doctor. He couldn't imagine that I didn't feel bad because I needed to receive two pints of blood immediately and more tests. Before I could turn around, I was in the hospital. I was told I had a tumor under my liver and needed an operation.

Following the operation, the words *not getting all the tumor, malignant cancer, the need to remove part of my small intestines,* and *treatment required* were what I heard from the doctor. These words hit my head and my heart.

With winter on the way, we decided to move to Colorado to be near our family. Shortly after we moved, my wife also was diagnosed with cancer. My family, golf buddies, and friends drove me more than 180 miles to the hospital in Denver for my treatments each Monday. The chemotherapy caused painful reactions. After a few rounds of chemotherapy, a day came when my spirits were so low that my zest for life was gone. I held a gun to my head to end all my misery. Just then, the words "that's not the way" came into my head. I believe the Good Lord stopped me, and I had a different feeling throughout the rest of my treatments. From that moment, I began to gain strength and believed there was some reason for me to go on.

How thankful I am that the rest of my 29 treatments went better. The care, understanding, and professionalism I experienced at the Denver Veteran's Hospital were outstanding. I know there was a jewel in the crown of hope for a better life.

Two years later, my wife passed away. I received a phone call from one of our friends who read the obituary in her Florida newspaper. She started writing notes of encouragement to me, and, would you believe, a year later we were married—on my 74th birthday! What a present! Since that time, I've become a Christian and am active in our church. I work two days a week as a gate attendant at the beach, line dance once a week, and golf two days a week. In December, my grandson and I played in the Father and Son Team Classic golf tournament at Pebble Beach, CA. We came in fifth place and I was the oldest of 200 participants. This year, I even made two holes in one! I'm blessed and thankful.

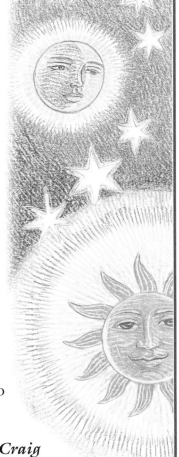

Dan Craig
Four-plus year cancer survivor
Florida

We've realized how much we care about and need each other—more than we possibly could imagine. With everything that has happened to us, our relationship as a family has never been stronger, and that strength grows each day.

Linda Allard
Part of a family fighting together
California

The Cancer Christmas

Cancer teaches a family how to react to the valleys in life.

My family story with the cancer experience began with my breast cancer diagnosis when I was 40 years old. I was working for a major airline carrier; my husband's business was thriving; and our children, ages 18, 14, and 9, were healthy and involved with school, swim team, tennis, and friends. Life was good!

We were determined to get through this cancer episode with very few real disruptions in our lives. When my oncologist tried to temper my optimistic attitude with realism, I replied, "Oh, but you don't know me!" We were open with the children concerning surgery, explaining mastectomy and chemotherapy (before the new antinausea medicine was available), hair loss, wigs, and my prosthesis. In fact, the children thought my prosthesis was especially neat.

"Pollyanna" should have been my middle name. As my treatments stretched into months, the toll of chemotherapy, nausea, vomiting, neutropenia, infections, stomatitis, and fatigue affected each of us. To make matters worse, we were in the midst of a terrible Midwest winter. Christmas was approaching. My life, which was already complicated by cancer treatments, now had the added dimension of snow, sleet, ice storms, and gray days. The cold and wind were bone-chilling. I often complained of not being able to get warm. I especially hated that cold prosthesis on chilly mornings. Life was hard! It seemed a continuous series of never-ending hurdles. Radiation therapy was still looming on the horizon.

Every mother wants Christmas to be special for her children, especially when faced with a life-threatening illness. Cancer should not be on a nine-year-old child's mind at this time of year. I was determined that we follow all of our family traditions. We purchased the gifts, including a waterbed for our youngest daughter. The cookies, tree, and dinner were just like our past family Christmases.

It is amazing how little things can bother you when you don't feel well. I awoke Christmas morning and the smell of the turkey that I had cooked overnight turned my stomach. The bedroom was freezing, the insides of the bedroom windows were covered with frost, there was not enough hot water for my shower, my church clothes didn't fit anymore, my head was cold, we were in danger of being late for church, and I couldn't find my prosthesis. I had lost my prosthesis before—left it inside my bra, in the clothes hamper, on the vanity, on a night table, and even on the floor. Searching for my prosthesis had become a family joke. This morning, however, it did not seem so funny. I was just about ready to stuff my bra with socks when I gave a yell, "Has anybody seen my breast?!"

My nine-year-old daughter came into the bedroom, angelic in her Christmas clothes. She explained that she knew how much I hated the cold prosthesis, so she had put it underneath the covers in her new waterbed so it would be warm for me this Christmas morning. As I hugged her, I realized how deeply cancer had affected my family. Even though life was hard right now, it was also very good!

On the way to church, we laughed. In the back of our minds was the uncertainty of future Christmases together. Cancer does that to a family. But cancer also can bring out the best qualities in a family, enriching an already loving marriage and preparing children for a life that isn't always picture-book perfect. Cancer teaches a family how to react to the valleys in life. Our family's cancer Christmas was in 1990.

Kathleen O'Sullivan, RN, BSN, ARNPS
Wife, mother, nurse, and breast cancer survivor
Florida

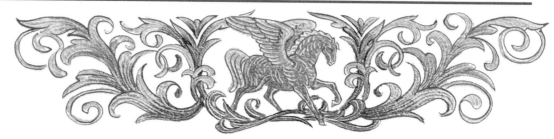

Camp CARE

*I just had to think positive thoughts and
look forward to being like I once was before.*

I was diagnosed with leukemia on my sixth birthday. It was a very difficult thing to deal with and brought a bunch of stress for my parents. It really hurt to walk along the street and hear someone talking or laughing at me. My hair fell out about five times because I had to take chemotherapy. I was in the hospital for months at a time—on Christmas for about two or three years, for all my family's birthdays, on Valentine's Day, etc. It was a really stressful thing to deal with. To tell you the truth, I really disliked my life at that time. I felt like it was my fault everything was happening the way it was. But deep down inside, I knew it was no one's fault. I just had to think positive thoughts and look forward to being like I was once before. I remember lying in the hospital bed with my parents talking, playing games, and just being a "special" family. It was so much fun to be that close to my loving parents.

My favorite nurse was a woman named Trisha. She is really sweet, caring, and very friendly. I see her about every year at Camp CARE. Camp CARE is a *wonderful* camp I attend every summer. It's held on Lake Lure. CARE stands for Cancer Ain't Really the End—and that statement is 100% true. I was six when I had cancer, and I am almost 15 now and I look healthier than ever. I have been in remission for almost five years. So all of you out there who have cancer, look for all of the positive things in life and everything will turn out for the better. Remember you are *special* people to me and surely to everyone else. You always will have a special place in my heart and just remember, I love you.

Crystal Quick
Leukemia survivor
North Carolina

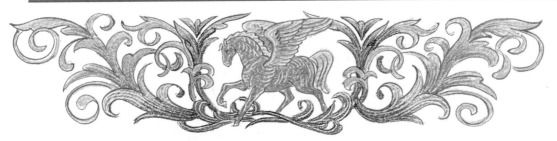

Reflections on Womanhood in the Face of Cancer

*It was time for me to redefine my view of
womanhood and the priorities in my life.*

At age 39, I had a toddler, a career, and a "bikini-cut" hysterectomy for early-stage cervical cancer. And life went on. Five years later, I was facing breast cancer. The scars were healing, but life was not going on just like before—not this time. As I stared into the mirror, I looked for Sandy, the woman. I saw baldness instead of stylish locks of hair, a flat chest with scars instead of full breasts. I was out of estrogen and into a larger dress size! It was time for me to redefine my view of womanhood and the priorities in my life. My husband, Nicholas, pointed out that my breasts and uterus had done their job well —just look at our precious, healthy daughter, Alexa. You know, he was right! Now I have short hair . . . it's fun and easy to care for. I'm working on my dress size, but I'm glad the baggy look is in style. I'm finding ways to cope with menopause and other side effects of the chemotherapy. It's nice to just relax and stroll along the beach. I took a break from work to spend more time with family, friends, and fellow cancer survivors who have all been so wonderful and supportive. Once again, I study my reflection in the mirror. I see a wife, a mother, a daughter, a sister. . . . I see a woman full of life. I see Sandy, a cancer survivor.

Sandy Von Staden
Two-year breast cancer survivor
Florida

*Don't worry until you have something to
worry about. Then, don't worry. Do
something about it!*

Gene Blumenschein
Five-year colon cancer survivor
Ohio

Now! Don't Wait!

*Times with family members are irreplaceable and the stuff
my happiness is made of. Now I try to make these opportunities
rather than wait for them to happen.*

I want to hang on to the feelings of my new life—it's a fresh start. I work at keeping these thoughts and feelings close to the surface of my mind, readily available when things don't go well.

Going through a bone marrow transplant in 1987 changed the way I look at my life. Of great importance to me now are my priorities: my family, expanding my interests now that I am retired, painting, travel, and helping others get through what I went through.

I'm spending time alone with each of our kids whenever possible. A year ago, our daughter and I spent a week together on Cape Cod, just the two of us. February: Cold, rainy, windswept—we loved it, and we decided to fit in a little time together alone, some-where—anywhere—each year.

Last summer, I went to Massachusetts to help one of our sons settle into his new apartment. We had great fun at the discounter's buying things he needed. He's a bachelor and lives like one. We had dinner together in the evenings and told each other how terrific we were to get such bargains. These times with family members are irreplaceable and the stuff my happiness is made of. Now I try to make these opportunities rather than wait for them to happen.

About the time I had my bone marrow transplant, Cleveland State University offered the "Project 60" program. This project allows anyone over 60 years old to take courses free of charge. I've been taking courses ever since—Chinese language, music appreciation, Mozart operas, religion courses, and, most important of all, painting. All my life, I've been looking at paintings. I taught high school art but have never painted. Looking back, I think I was afraid to paint—it meant too much to me. I could never produce a painting I would like. But there is something about the cancer experience, and the transplant in particular, that shaved away the veneer of my inhibition. What really matters became obvious to me. I keep three big words pasted on the inside of my brain: NOW! DON'T WAIT!

As a volunteer on the bone marrow unit, I am acutely reminded of the discomfort, fear, and just plain boredom I encountered while undergoing my transplant back in 1987. I understand what the patients are going through and I empathize. As I began volunteering, I had hoped to encourage patients through the tough times of treatment. I have learned, however, that I am the one who benefits most from attending these support groups. The patients' courage, optimism, and mutual support are inspiring. As I watch the protocols become more streamlined, how can I not be optimistic?

I had such a fine support system when I went through the procedure. Our daughter, Chandlee, found out about transplants at a medical school lecture. Our son Jeff transferred his residency to Cleveland so he could help me get through it. Our other son, Mitch, taught me guided imagery, and my husband visited me every day and was remarkable in his thoughtfulness. I am very lucky.

All these experiences have made me want to hang onto the feelings of my new life—it's a fresh start. I work at keeping these thoughts and feelings close to the surface of my mind, readily available when things do not go well. In Bob Woodward's recent book, *The Choice,* he quotes Elizabeth Dole: "I've had to learn that dependence is a good thing. Then, when I've used up my own resources, when I can't control things and make them come out my way, I'm willing to trust God with the outcome." She said so eloquently what I feel.

Pid Dickey
Ten-year bone marrow transplant survivor
Ohio

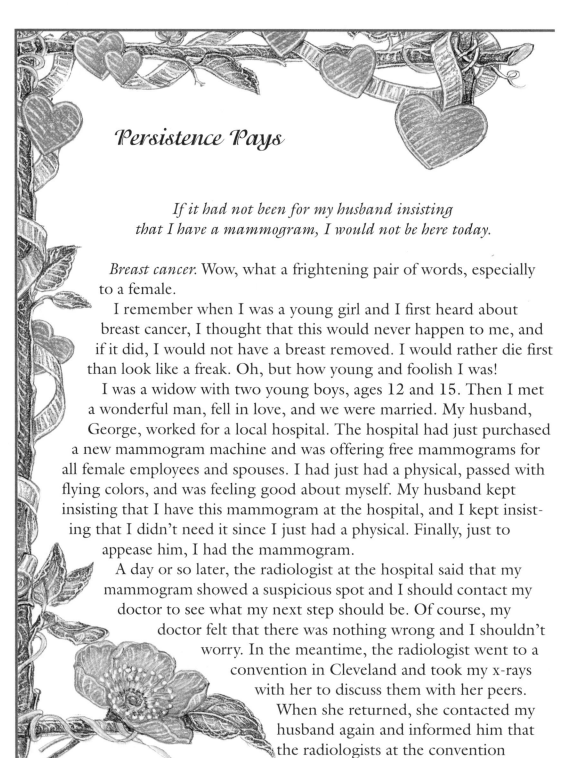

Persistence Pays

*If it had not been for my husband insisting
that I have a mammogram, I would not be here today.*

Breast cancer. Wow, what a frightening pair of words, especially to a female.

I remember when I was a young girl and I first heard about breast cancer, I thought that this would never happen to me, and if it did, I would not have a breast removed. I would rather die first than look like a freak. Oh, but how young and foolish I was!

I was a widow with two young boys, ages 12 and 15. Then I met a wonderful man, fell in love, and we were married. My husband, George, worked for a local hospital. The hospital had just purchased a new mammogram machine and was offering free mammograms for all female employees and spouses. I had just had a physical, passed with flying colors, and was feeling good about myself. My husband kept insisting that I have this mammogram at the hospital, and I kept insisting that I didn't need it since I just had a physical. Finally, just to appease him, I had the mammogram.

A day or so later, the radiologist at the hospital said that my mammogram showed a suspicious spot and I should contact my doctor to see what my next step should be. Of course, my doctor felt that there was nothing wrong and I shouldn't worry. In the meantime, the radiologist went to a convention in Cleveland and took my x-rays with her to discuss them with her peers. When she returned, she contacted my husband again and informed him that the radiologists at the convention thought it looked suspicious. Again, I confronted my doctor who, at this time, decided to send me out of town to another physician. He checked the x-rays and said he felt 99% sure it was nothing, but to be sure he would do a biopsy.

After a few days, we went back for the results. I could tell as soon as I went into the examining room that all was not well. It was *cancer*. I had a mastectomy and reconstruction. Nothing was found in the lymph nodes the surgeon removed, nor in the surrounding tissues. I had no radiation follow-up.

I am writing this more than 10 years later. If it had not been for my husband, George, insisting that I have a mammogram, and the radiologist pursuing the x-rays, I strongly feel that I would not be here today.

One more thing—I certainly do not feel like a freak. I feel truly blessed.

Brigitte Brant Diez
Ten-year breast cancer survivor
Ohio

One night, we were sitting on the couch coloring in a "Snow White and the Seven Dwarfs" coloring book that my cousin had sent to help pass the time. My mother spotted Dopey, his bald head covered by a cap, and said, "Hey, that's me!" Dopey became her mascot from then on. My mother recently celebrated her first year of being cancer-free, and she is back to dancing several nights a week. We still have a two-foot-tall Dopey in our living room to remind us of the positive attitude and sense of humor that she maintained through it all.

Leslie Bates
Daughter of ovarian cancer survivor
California

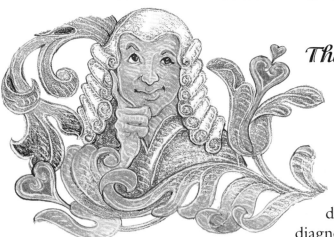

The Wedding

What if someone hugged me at the wedding and walked away with my wig on their watch?

Eight weeks before my daughter's wedding, I was diagnosed with breast cancer. My doctor informed me that the treatment would consist of chemotherapy, surgery, bone marrow transplantation, and radiation, and we were to start immediately.

I needed to rearrange my schedule, but most of all I needed a plan. I took my two best friends wig shopping with me, and for a couple hours that afternoon I was a blonde, redhead, and even "Cher." I settled for a brunette wig that looked just like my disappearing hair. It was actually a fun afternoon. I have the greatest friends!

A few weeks later, my list consisted of unusual concerns. My wig slid sideways one day when I put my purse strap on my shoulder, so I discovered skull caps and two-sided tape. But what if someone hugged me at the wedding and walked away with my wig on their watch? My eyelashes were history (as were my eyebrows), so should I try the false ones? What if I cry and they fall off? I decided to forego the false lashes. I also had to deal with hot flashes, a puffy face, and shoes that no longer fit (because of my swollen feet). But what a small price to pay. . . .

It seemed so fitting to have a wedding that day. The air was clean and crisp, and the sun was shining so beautifully on all the vibrant colors of autumn. The wedding was perfect, and my daughter, radiant! I had enough energy to really enjoy the day. I felt so very lucky to be alive. Oh, and my wig stayed on.

Chris Richards
Two-year breast cancer survivor
California

Chapter 4

Personal Connections: A Guiding Light Through the Cancer Experience

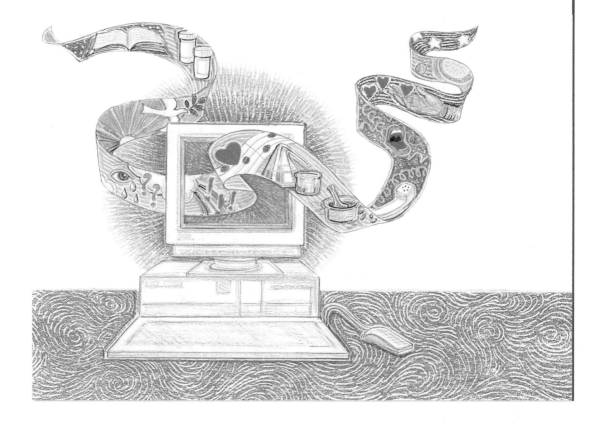

My Seventh Friend

He left, and I felt loved!

My first friend came and expressed his shock by saying, "I can't believe that you have cancer. I always thought you were so active and healthy."

He left, and I felt alienated and somehow very "different."

My second friend came and brought me information about a variety of cancer treatments. He said, "Whatever you do, don't take chemotherapy. It's a poison!"

He left, and I felt scared and confused.

My third friend came and tried to answer my "whys" with the statement, "Perhaps God is disciplining you for some sin in your life."

He left, and I felt guilty.

My fourth friend came and told me, "If your faith is just great enough, God will heal you."

He left, and I felt that my faith must be inadequate.

My fifth friend came and told me to remember that "all things work together for good."

He left, and I felt angry.

My sixth friend never came at all.

I felt sad and alone.

My seventh friend came and held my hand and said, "I care, I'm here, I want to help you through this."

He left, and I felt loved!

Linda Mae Richardson
Sixteen-year melanoma survivor
Kansas

I became a witness to the beautiful art of friendship. People opened their hearts to me, expressed their feelings, and carried me through treatment with their prayers, love, and affection.

Patricia L. Kinney
Breast cancer and bone marrow transplant
survivor, a.k.a. "Alive and well!"
Arizona

LEAPS and Bounds

Lou turned a negative personal experience into a positive outcome. She is a survivor who has helped hundreds of other people who have suffered this profound physical change.

Lou Keyes' experience is a classic example of a silver lining. She always has been a dynamic, motivated, and physically and socially active person. She believes in maintaining a good, healthy life-style to stay well. Her endeavors seemed successful until February 18, 1986, when she learned that she had a malignant bone tumor at the top of her right femur, into the pelvis. The only way to ensure that she would have a fighting chance to beat this disease was to undergo radical amputation of her right leg and the entire right pelvis.

To most people, coping with such an immense change in body image would be overwhelming. However, Lou turned a very negative personal experience into a positive outcome. Almost immediately after her recovery from the surgery, she formed an organization for other amputees called Lower Extremity Amputees Providing Support—LEAPS. Originally, Lou was the only member, but, mainly through word of mouth, the group has grown to approximately 250 members.

LEAPS offers monthly support meetings, newsletters, social activities, telephone contacts that are followed up with personal visits to amputees, and resources for prostheses and other supplies. By offering ongoing support, Lou's group helps its members cope with a drastic change in body image and adjust to the impact it has on activities of daily living. Lou always is there for any member who needs assistance and support. She is a survivor who has helped, and will continue to help, hundreds of other people who have suffered a profound physical change, either through a surgical amputation, accident, or birth defect. Anyone wishing more information about LEAPS can contact Lou at 816-361-3206.

Dorothy A. Bailey, RN
Nurse and friend of Lou Keyes, cancer survivor
Missouri

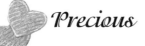

Precious

Cancer separates us from other people. We hear our meters ticking.

Nobody chooses it. Yet, it provides an opportunity—a perspective many people achieve only on their deathbed. This separates us from others because we hear our meters ticking. Rather than lament decisions, we can reframe our lives. We know that our lives may be downsized. We set new priorities.

Joining this involuntary sisterhood took me back to regular meetings with other women, meetings of the '60s and the '70s. As before, sharing thoughts and emotions sheds clarity on individual situations and options. We gain strength by processing our terror, fear, ignorance, and knowledge. We laugh and cry to heal ourselves.

Our meetings are a refuge, a psychological free zone unlike other hours in our days. In group we don't have to coddle the fears of others. We don't have to pretend it doesn't linger in our minds. We understand us.

My most intense hours are those with my group, with other women struggling to make informed decisions and to live through adversity with dignity. We help each other cope with doctors, employers, friends, lovers, and family. What's the answer to "Mommie, are you gonna die?"

A year later, my existence has different rhythms and melodies. Although each of us navigates her own hurricanes, I believe that part of me lives the life of every woman in our group. We are community. We choose to live well and to be present. We appreciate every day. We know that every one of us is precious.

Karen Folger Jacobs, PhD
Writer and breast cancer survivor
California

Compassionate Coworkers

*The love and support I have received from everyone
I know will carry me through this.*

In January of 1996, I accepted a position as a legal secretary at the Boston law firm of Rackemann, Sawyer and Brewster. In June of 1996, I was diagnosed with a very rare form of cancer originating in my salivary gland that very quickly spread to my lungs. I had two operations, one on my neck to remove the original tumor and one on my chest. My prognosis was bleak: 6–18 months to live.

I left work in July on long-term disability status with no idea whether I would ever return. Not long afterwards, I received a letter and a card telling me that approximately 50 people from the firm had donated both their personal and vacation days, which allowed me to collect 100% of my salary up to the end of December 1996. I was required to be out of work continuously for six months before I could collect long-term disability payments. This gift of donated time was truly overwhelming. These beautiful people continue to call and send cards and good wishes. I am a single parent raising my son and daughter alone, and it has always been a struggle to survive.

In September of 1996, the managing partner of the firm called to say that the firm wanted to do something more to make our lives easier. They arranged to pay our heating bills for the coming winter! Heating a home in the Northeast is very expensive in the winter. I was totally overwhelmed by all this goodness.

I have received two three-day treatments of chemotherapy, four weeks apart, and my doctor told me that one of the larger tumors in my lung is gone! I have a strong faith in God and the power of the mind to overcome adversity. I believe that I will recover from this illness. All pain is an avenue toward growth. My pain has shown me that the love and support I have received from everyone I know will carry me through this. I will be one of the miracles. After all, I need to go back to work at Rackemann, Sawyer and Brewster because they are holding my job open for me!

Virginia M. Dexter
Mother and cancer survivor
Massachusetts

World Turned Upside Down

Friendships are strengthened as we walk through the valley of cancer.

I never really understood what it meant to have your world turned "upside down" until July 31, 1980. I will never forget the doctor's words: "I'm sorry, but you have cancer." He went on to explain that I had malignant melanoma that had spread to my lymph system. I was in shock. He told me that he knew of no effective treatment. He referred me to M.D. Anderson Cancer Center in Houston, TX, where I underwent surgery, radiation, and chemotherapy. Because I had more than 50 malignant lymph nodes involved, my prognosis seemed grim.

I doubt that any family is ever prepared to deal with a serious illness such as cancer. Mine was certainly no exception. Although death is not something anyone likes to talk about, my illness brought us face-to-face with that possibility. We discovered that voicing our fears helped lessen them.

It has been 15 years since my last treatment, and my tests remain clear. I am filled with gratitude for this time that I have been given. After treatment, I wanted to forget about my cancer. However, I had a greater desire to reach out and help other patients with this disease. In 1984, I became involved with a cancer support group called Victory in the Valley. This group provides a safe and caring environment in which to share our hopes and fears. Friendships are strengthened as we walk through the valley of cancer.

I realize that tomorrow is always uncertain, but each time I hug my family and hold my new granddaughter, I whisper a quiet prayer of thanks to God, who has helped us through it all!

Linda Mae Richardson
Sixteen-year melanoma survivor
Kansas

Returning the Blessing

Volunteering to spread a message of hope and encouragement was a wonderful opportunity.

I was diagnosed with lung cancer in 1985. My surgeon was able to remove the center section of my right lung where the cancer was contained. Because there was no lymph node involvement, my oncologist decided that chemotherapy and radiation were not required.

In 1986, I became a cancer hotline phone volunteer. I felt blessed to be able to help other patients with cancer and their families. Volunteering to spread a message of hope and encouragement was a wonderful opportunity.

In 1989, an answering service offered to direct all hotline calls after office hours and on weekends to my home. Thanks to their efforts, each year I talk with approximately 800 patients with cancer, their families, and friends from all over the world.

The joy, pain, and sorrow I share with these callers will live with me forever. I thank God each day for this opportunity. It is my way of returning the blessing of being cancer-free for 11 years.

Rosemary Sill
Eleven-year lung cancer survivor
Missouri

It was almost like I was given breast cancer in order to help other women. Breast cancer can be a positive experience if you make the most of a bad situation. Life goes on after cancer—sometimes it's even a better life!

Kimberly A. Stoliker
Four-year breast cancer survivor
New York

Living With Loneliness

"One is the loneliest number that you'll ever know. Two can be as bad as one. It's the loneliest number since the number one."

These are the opening lyrics of a song made popular by the pop group Three Dog Night in the early '70s. The great philosophers and poets of ancient Greece couldn't have said it any better. We all think we have experienced loneliness. The teenage girl is crying in her room after breaking up with her first love, the young boy is sitting in the back seat of a police cruiser after being caught speeding, and the divorced wife is looking at the empty kitchen table on her anniversary date. These are truly moments of despair, but no one knows loneliness like a person fighting cancer. The physical pain we may feel in our bodies is nothing compared to the pain we so often feel in our hearts and souls.

I remember, during my own treatment, going to the supermarket one day with my wife. I had been neutropenic (low white blood cell count) for several weeks and had been confined to my home. A trip to the grocery store was my big day out. I remember walking down the aisles of food, looking at the many different colors and shapes of containers. They all appeared different that day. I saw them in a new context. I remember watching the people. An old, retired couple shopped together—the aging husband pushing the cart, his gray-haired wife squinting to read her shopping list and double-checking her coupons. The young mother struggled—one child was fussing in her shopping cart and the other was sorting through the cereal aisle trying to find the best treasure. The college student cruised around with his cart full of beer, beans, and franks. The red-headed housewife carefully checked the vegetables while the blonde, stately madam inspected the bananas. Numerous human creatures went through the ritual of "gathering" while others practiced the ancient rite of "hunting." All were obtaining food for their families. Loneliness—I had been isolated so long that even a trip to the grocery store now opened new realizations.

At the end of the canned goods aisle, I encountered an old family friend. "I wonder how Fred and his wife are doing?" I thought, but by the time I worked my way to the end of the aisle, he was gone. Humans are such predictable creatures. Fred doesn't know how to handle my disease. I know he wanted to talk with me, but he didn't know what to say or do. So, he decided that the best way to handle this confrontation was to avoid me completely. Fred had never felt comfortable enough with my disease to come and visit me in the hospital, nor did he call me at home. And now—not on purpose—he physically deserted me. This happens every day, in every community, in every home where a person faces cancer. Dealing with situations like this is what Gilda's Club is all about—getting rid of loneliness, despair, and melancholy. Gilda's Club, a cancer support program created in memory of comedian Gilda Radner, is a place to go, a place to talk with other people with cancer, and a place to do things. It's a place where family members of patients with cancer can talk and interact with other families facing the same ordeals. Gilda's Club is a place to gain knowledge, a place to gain strength, and a place to cry. Gilda's Clubs are popping up across the United States. Please support them.

James W. Pleasant
Bone marrow transplant survivor
Ohio

At first, I felt it would be uncomfortable to go to a support group, but later I changed my mind and decided to try it. Now I participate in two groups. It has helped me feel less alone. I have met some wonderful women who will be my friends for life.

Kathie Gepfert, RN
Breast cancer survivor
Colorado

CyberSisters

*Just reach out, turn on your computer,
and open up a whole new world!*

My husband and I waited for what seemed like hours for the doctor to give us my biopsy results. We were the only ones left in the office after closing hours. The doctor walked right out into the waiting room and sat next to us and said those dreaded words, "Well, I am sorry to say, it is cancer." I finally knew for the first time what it meant to have the wind knocked out of your sails! I could not breathe. My husband, Denny, was as shocked as I was. I could see that he and the doctor were talking, yet, I was just sitting there in stunned disbelief.

I was very fortunate in that I had a multilevel system of support. I attended a formal support group at Good Samaritans' Cancer Institute, which offered not only group discussions but also, on occasion, guest speakers who were helpful in a variety of ways. As a patient at St. Mary's-Good Samaritan, I also had the opportunity to meet twice monthly with a wonderful oncology counselor, Patricia Liebman, LCSW. Without her help, I would not have obtained the level of growth that I have. She led me to my "fantabulous" oncologist, Dr. Elizabeth McKeen. Both of them are a blessing that has come from my cancer experience. They are my angels!

My younger sister also was a wonderful supporter. As a trained pastoral counselor, she had many tools to assist me. She was diagnosed with breast cancer four years ago. Even with this family history of cancer, I never thought it would happen to me. Why me? Why not me?! I was totally shell-shocked, and then another bomb landed. My dear mother also was diagnosed with cancer. My "Why me?" turned into "Why us?"

My life changed so fast after my cancer diagnosis. After the hectic and painful time of making all the quick decisions and planning and undergoing operations, including reconstruction, I found myself sitting at home still in a state of shock. I desperately needed to talk with someone who had gone through this dark and lonely forest before me. I was looking for someone who knew what to expect next and how long the pain would last. In addition, I had a hundred other questions. I spent many hours just weeping. Just as I thought I had everything under control, out of the blue, tears would stream down and wash my cheeks. Sometimes they still do, but now I know that is normal. At the time, I thought I was going crazy, ripping apart at my new tattered seams.

My husband had just bought a new computer. Being a mom, a grandmother of seven, and a stay-at-home wife, I hardly knew how to turn it on. But something told me to search for other women who were in the same boat. I'd hoped to find someone who had chosen a mastectomy with immediate reconstruction. I saw the screen flash "search topic" and typed in "breast cancer." I would have used the word "survivor" also, but, at that point, the word had no meaning for me. Well, much to my surprise, up popped a long list of women. It was joy and sadness all rolled into one. So many had walked my walk—women of all ages, races, sizes, and faiths. Women from every corner of the map.

I then discovered that you could pull up profiles of the women on the list. I was guided by my higher power to two women's names. I sent Ginger and Perry e-mail, asking if either would be interested in "chatting" with me because I wanted to talk with someone else who had this feared disease. Much to my delight and surprise, they both wrote back very encouraging words. For the first time, I felt that someone really understood where I was coming from. It was a miracle for me.

Since that first e-mail, which I sent in January of 1996, our group has grown to a dozen wonderful and spiritual women. A braver group of women you have never seen! Computer support groups can be developed and customized individually. You are in control of how you set up your own support system. Some people are more comfortable with just one computer buddy.

Every day, I look forward to turning on my computer. I know that someone will have sent an encouraging word or positive affirmation by way of e-mail. Or, maybe someone else has reached out and asked for help because the roller coaster of life after cancer has gotten her down.

At times, I am able to offer an encouraging word to help another back up the hill.

After a diagnosis of cancer, survivors get double vision. We are glad to have found each other but sad that our numbers are so large. I am thrilled to know that I can give support to others who need it, yet I'm sad to have experienced this disease. I have received so much sustenance and love from these women that it brings tears to my eyes. In addition, chatting about the cancer experience on-line has given me the opportunity to share my belief in God and to offer help to others. This opportunity gave me back my self-esteem. I know I really do make a difference and that people really do care!

So, if any of you are too distanced from a support group or you prefer or need to stay at home, just reach out, turn on your computer, and make daily connections with new, understanding friends. Let the people out there know who you are. Share your profile. I assure you that it will make a difference in their lives as well as your own. This has opened up a whole new world for me. I have been truly blessed with my new friends. It has turned my scars into stars! I even had a great big hug ((((((WANDA)))))) on my computer when I found out I needed another biopsy in my left breast. We share stories, poems, prayers, and even a few jokes. We weep together, and we laugh together, but, most of all, we share a sisterhood of love, compassion, and support. And we know that we really can survive!

Wanda Deems (wandawell@aol.com)
Mother of four, proud grandmother of seven,
and breast cancer survivor
Florida

I see and hear of so much need in dealing with cancer. If we all band together and support each other, perhaps we can offer some hope.

Patti Lewis
Writer, liturgical designer, clergy spouse, and
two-year breast cancer survivor
Arizona

The Spider Man

*He stated that his radiation marks made him
the true Spider Man!*

While in graduate school in Florida, I volunteered at
the American Cancer Society's Winn Dixie Hope Lodge.
This was a hotel where patients with cancer and their families could
stay while receiving treatment. While there, I met Brian, a four-year-
old with bone cancer who was receiving treatment at a local medical
center. He was full of energy and excited about being in a new city.
He was scheduled for seven weeks of radiation treatments. Yet, he
was most excited about Halloween, which was only two days
away. He had his Spider Man costume ready and was all set to
trick or treat. Unfortunately, the next morning he awoke with a
$104°$ temperature and was admitted to the hospital for a week. He
missed Halloween and was very disappointed.

The other patients at the Hope Lodge felt for Brian. Upon his
return to the lodge, they hosted a belated Halloween party for him.
Patients, families, volunteers, and Brian's physicians were there. He was
so surprised and happy! He didn't even put on his Spider Man mask—
he said that his radiation marks made him the true Spider Man! To this
day, this was the happiest Halloween I have ever had. It was the most
touching for Brian.

Kimberly G. Bogart, RN
Oncology nurse for eight years
Georgia

Most of my memories now aren't real clear;
That year as a patient was not my career.
But nurses, their talents and comforting ways
Will live in my mind all the rest of my days.

Mary Greene Lamb
Breast cancer survivor
Arizona

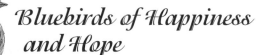

Bluebirds of Happiness and Hope

It never ceases to amaze me how the word "cancer" changes lives so quickly and dramatically!

St. Thomas Hospital in Nashville, TN, teamed up with the Telephone Pioneers (the Retired Communication Workers of America) and started Camp Bluebird. This camp is for cancer survivors, whether they have survived for one day or many years. They are *all* survivors!

Camp Bluebird offers a rustic, three-day retreat for individuals who are battling or have survived cancer. The camp is located on a beautiful, woodsy site in central Tennessee and is managed by volunteers, some of whom are nurses. It provides a time and place for patients with cancer to come together and share their concerns, fears, and hopes for the future. Each camper is assigned to a counselor who has been trained to provide education and support. The name "Camp Bluebird" originated from the Blue South Pioneers' project of preserving bluebirds in the Southeast. Each camper has the opportunity to build a birdhouse to assist the Pioneers in this project.

The concept of Camp Bluebird was developed by cancer survivor Louis Josof of Saint Vincent's Hospital in Birmingham, AL. Gloria Cherry, RN, a former St. Vincent's nurse, implemented the idea of the camp for St. Thomas Hospital. John Tighe, president and chief executive officer of St. Thomas Hospital, described Camp Bluebird as "a place where miracles happen. It is a place where people are understood and get empathy, not sympathy. It is a place where you can laugh and cry in the same breath. It also is one of the best things St. Thomas has ever done to live out its mission."

The camp provides a haven for listening, learning, sharing, and caring. Campers analyze their life-style adjustments in living with cancer. Families learn how to give and receive support. They also learn how to assess and meet nonmedical needs. Healthcare professionals provide information on nutrition and how to manage cancer treatments and their side effects. While arts and crafts provide creative outlets, skits, challenges, and bonding discussions offer emotional support for all participants. Camp Bluebird helps patients with cancer take control of their lives.

The funds for Camp Bluebird are generated by a dogwood Christmas tree in the lobby of St. Thomas that is decorated with blue lights and wooden bluebirds. The bluebirds, which are made by a local craftsman, are sold for $15 each in honor or memory of a loved one and are placed on the beautiful tree. The bluebirds symbolize happiness, inspiration, and hope. Though the bluebird is quite small, it is very powerful.

I am grateful to be an oncology nurse, cancer survivor, and volunteer for this project. I am not the same person that I was when I first heard the word "cancer." I was 27 years old then. I am now 51. I no longer take anything for granted. It is hard to describe, but since my cancer diagnosis, I am different. Yes, cancer changes the lives of everyone involved—not just at that time, but forever. I feel I have a message I can share with other people who have cancer because I have been there. I know what it is like firsthand. For me, it has been a positive experience. I have gained so much. I am thankful for life. I live one moment at a time. I know in my heart that God will bless us all on this journey called life. He will see us through.

Rosemary Talbott, LPN
Mother of four and soon-to-be-grandmother of five,
hospital chaplain, oncology licensed practical nurse,
and cancer survivor
Tennessee

My condition has led me to much-improved family relationships; it has made me more tolerant, more compassionate, more understanding, and more spiritual. I have a greater appreciation for life and humor.

Martin Kobrin
Prostate cancer survivor
Florida

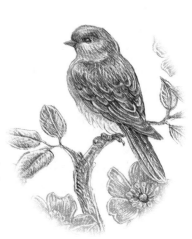

She Found Her True Calling

She truly exemplifies oncology nursing.

"Your hair will grow back! After all, mine did . . . and doesn't it look great?"

Whenever I hear Sue explain the side effects of chemotherapy to her patients, I have to smile. You see, Sue has only been a nurse for three years. Being a wife, mother, and lawyer came first. Then, one morning about six years ago, her life changed drastically. Severe fatigue forced her to visit her doctor. Several days later, Sue was diagnosed with acute myelogenous leukemia.

Her treatment began immediately. Once she entered remission, she received an allogeneic bone marrow transplant. The transplant was not successful, and a subsequent autologous transplant followed. Then, after several months of infections, she achieved remission once again!

Sue was very thankful to the caring, supportive nurses who helped her through those long months. She really admired their dedication.

When Sue returned to work at her law office, she had a conversation with a close colleague. He said, "You are a great lawyer. You give a lot of yourself. But I can tell you are not truly happy here. What better time to change careers than now?"

Soon after their conversation, Sue enrolled in nursing school. Upon graduation, she started working on a cardiac unit. However, her real goal was oncology. As soon as a position was available, she began to work on my oncology unit.

Sue loves working at the bedside. She frequently is found sitting beside a patient, holding his or her hand, and offering words of support and comfort, as well as providing hugs to patients, family members, and staff. If she thinks it might be helpful, she will share some of her own experiences with cancer. She supports patients in making decisions about their treatments. Follow-up visits and phone calls come naturally to Sue.

Sue is a member of the Oncology Nursing Society (ONS) and the ONS Chicago Chapter. This past year, Sue received her BSN and became certified in medical-surgical, critical care, and oncology nursing. She currently is working toward her master's degree in oncology nursing.

Patients, families, and the staff love Sue. She truly exemplifies oncology nursing.

Linda A. Skrzypczynski, RN, C, OCN®
Oncology nurse
Illinois

On my last night in that ward, my nurse came at the end of her shift to wish me well. I was so weak from pain medication and exhaustion that I couldn't even respond. I wish she could know how much her words meant to me.

David Stanley
Testicular cancer survivor
California

I am fine now. I hope I will be able to help someone else, as so many have helped me. I learned to live one day at a time and consider each day and each person to be very precious.

Frances Austin
Mother, grandmother, great-grandmother, and survivor of colon cancer
Tennessee

I urge all women to be aware of themselves. Always check on things that don't seem normal. You don't have to be afraid. There are people out there who can help you get through having breast cancer.

Sheryl Hawkins
Two-and-one-half-year breast cancer survivor
California

From Victim to Victor

Healing means more than physical health. It is also a continuous journey toward hope and peace of mind.

Things happen. Bad things happen. And when they happen to you, people call you a victim. I remember all too well when I became a cancer victim. At first, I was afraid because the word *cancer* is like some monster ready to grab you in the dark. A few weeks later, I came to hate the word *victim* even more because of what it meant. When I became a victim, I became helpless. And everyone knows, bad things happen to victims. Then, one day, I just decided I didn't like my assigned role. I was not going to play the victim any more. I learned an important lesson. It's my body, and no one cares about it as much as I do.

Shortly after major surgery, which confirmed the diagnosis of a later-stage ovarian cancer, I read a magazine article that said I had a 20% chance to live for a few years—if I was lucky. I cried and cried and cried some more, and then I threw the magazine across the room. Wow, did I ever feel better! Not only did anger release much of my bottled-up negative emotions, but it also was extremely energizing.

With the diagnosis of cancer and its accompanying emotional panic, I needed something to help with my depression and anxiety. I couldn't sleep, eat, or think. I was far from being rational! This certainly was no way to be making decisions. Although I feared ridicule from my healthcare providers, I asked for help and found that they were wondering when I was going to request assistance. They were expecting it and, contrary to my expectations, did not think less of me for the request. After that, I spent less time and anxiety over decisions that involved asking for help.

In the months after initial diagnosis and surgery, I read what I could about the type of cancer I had and its treatment. (It was never "my" cancer, as I never wanted it to own me, even if, at times, it felt like it did.) Our bodies are all different, and nobody reacts exactly the same to the same treatment. There are no absolutes with cancer treatment.

The effects of this disease on my family were disastrous. I felt guilty for raising my daughter's genetic health status into a "high risk" category. We all stopped laughing just when we needed humor the most. We had to force ourselves to seek humor. A dose of Erma Bombeck, Bill

Cosby, or the Three Stooges was far tastier than any dose of cod liver oil!

It was easy to stop talking to family and friends. I didn't want to tell them just how bad I felt physically and emotionally, and they didn't want to add to my burden by telling me everything they were thinking. The ensuing silence only worsened until we developed the art of "selective" sharing and listening.

But, oh, how I needed to communicate with another survivor of the same type of cancer! When I couldn't find one through a "grapevine" search, I thought there were no survivors. I wasn't sure I would find group meetings beneficial even if I did find others who had the same kind of cancer that I had. I found one long-term survivor through the Anderson Network (affiliated with M.D. Anderson Cancer Center in Houston, TX). Discovering her lit a candle of hope for me.

Realizing networking brought positive results, I placed an ad for "Contact with someone with same diagnosis" in the *Networker,* the newsletter of the National Coalition for Cancer Survivorship. Within a few days, I heard from 10 women from all over the country. The joy I felt from knowing that there were survivors of my type of cancer was, and still is, invigorating. What a bonfire of hope! We wrote and called each other often. A few months later, I found myself passing tips from one woman to another—like a wheel's center. So, on Halloween in 1993, with nothing more than a "wing and a prayer," I started the newsletter *CONVERSATIONS! The Newsletter for Women Who Are Fighting Ovarian Cancer.* Although the title seems a bit long, it is accurate. Those who are diagnosed with cancer will fight, in one way or another, cancer's effects on their body and soul for the rest of their lives. However, we are *not* victims, and we are *not* patients. We are women *first*—then we are women fighting cancer.

In the three-and-one-half years since the first issue was printed, the newsletter *CONVERSATIONS!* has become a supportive network for 1,000 women all over the United States and several foreign countries. Although we are in different stages of treatment, we have all discovered the strength that lies in knowing others have gone before us. No longer do we have to reinvent the wheel when there is a problem, as someone else already has experienced that problem and found solutions. When we pool our solutions, the answers are richer. For those who are not comfortable in formal groups, our network is a healthy form of support that is just as useful. What the future holds—for us as individuals, for the network, or for the newsletter—is uncertain, but for today it is helpful to me and others, burning brightly in the night.

Through it all, I have learned that "healing" means much more than physical health. Healing is a continuous journey toward Peace of mind and Hope for the next good moment. While cancer still lurks as a specter in the dark, I know this moment must be lived to the fullest. The *CONVERSA-TIONS!* newsletter motto, "Celebrating Life Today!" also has become my creed. Today, with all its dark and bright corners, must be savored and celebrated. After all, isn't this why we fight cancer so hard?

It hasn't been easy to change myself from victim to victor. Sometimes the progress backward is more visible than the progress forward. As I write this, on the fifth anniversary of my diagnosis, I know that if I can just enjoy whatever today has in store and keep facing forward, I am the victor!

CONVERSATIONS! The Newsletter for Women Who Are Fighting Ovarian Cancer is published monthly. The newsletter is free, but donations of about $20 per year to defray costs are gladly accepted. The focus of the newsletter is printed at the top of each issue: Caring, Sharing, Hoping, Healing, Helping, Coping, and "Humoring." It includes practical hints, inspirations, the latest research on prevention and treatment, book reviews, resources for help, and current events. (See the resource list at the back of this book for ordering information.)

Cindy H. Melancon
Five-year ovarian cancer survivor and thriver,
celebrating life today!
Texas

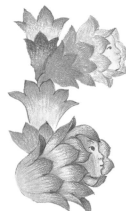

The cancer experience deepened Shirley's faith, enriched her life, and made her appreciate her loved ones even more. She felt that she met some wonderful people during her cancer experience. She just could not imagine not knowing them.

Linda Battiato, RN, MSN, OCN®
Oncology nurse
Indiana

Chance Encounters

Today, I continue to reach out to hold the hands of others with cancer knowing that our shared journeys bind us for life.

As we walk through life, our chance encounters must be treasured because they are often such defining moments in our lives. I'd like to share one of my special encounters.

During the course of my chemotherapy treatments leading to a stem cell transplant for breast cancer, I ventured into a movie theater. My hairless head was bedecked in a floppy hat, and my chemotherapy pump was around my waist. Waiting in the lobby for the movie to begin, I glanced around the room. A father and his teenage daughter sat along a wall. She wore a floppy hat on top of her hairless head; I did not see her chemotherapy pump. "Did you buy the hat at the same store as I did?" I asked. Her father smiled, and we engaged in a conversation. As we talked, the girl silently reached out and held my hand. It was warm and comforting. I asked her a question. She didn't answer, and, to my surprise, she released my hand to dart behind her father. Her father whispered that she was autistic. As I continued to talk to her father, she again reached out and held my hand. We stayed silently locked together until it was time to take our seats.

Throughout my course of treatments and until this day, I still feel her small hand in mine. It is a constant reminder of the strength within us. Today, I continue to reach out to hold the hands of others with cancer knowing that our shared journeys bind us for life.

Phyllis Katz
Breast cancer survivor, founder of
Legal Information Network for Cancer
Virginia

I feel I have been given a new life. I hope I live it well, using all I've learned to grow personally and to reach out to others in a meaningful way.

Jean Loving, RN
Hospice/oncology volunteer and
four-year breast cancer survivor
North Carolina

To My Friend

Just be yourself, be near, and persevere with me.

I know this word *cancer* is frightening to you. It is to me also. . . .

You ask what you can do for me. There are many things, but perhaps the most important are these.

Please do not stay away because of fear. I'm afraid also. I need you near to know that I'm not alone.

There are times when I will want to talk about my cancer—sometimes not.

But, most of all, just be yourself, be near, and persevere with me.

I know it will not always be easy for you, but I thank you for caring and for being my friend!

Linda Mae Richardson
Sixteen-year melanoma survivor
Kansas

By making yourself available and being open with your struggle, the people around you have the opportunity to learn to take their own lives one moment at a time. Being aware of the briefness of life, you are allowed to breathe deeply the moment that is. I think it is sometimes harder to be the one who loves the patient than to be the patient. The role of "just standing by" is a difficult one. I realize what a gift it was to others when I permitted them to assist me. Preparing a meal, washing clothes, car pooling, sending a card—all of these tangible signs of love and intention connected us together.

Libbie Kerr
Three-year breast cancer survivor
Ohio

Victory in the Valley

Good things can come from some of life's most difficult journeys.

In June of 1982, while preparing to go on a much-needed vacation, Lois Thomi discovered a red spot on the side of her breast. Not wanting it to interfere with her trip, she decided to visit her doctor to make sure it was nothing serious. After a series of tests, she found herself having a breast biopsy rather than a vacation. The results showed that Lois had inflammatory carcinoma of the breast. She was told that her prognosis was very poor. After undergoing a year of chemotherapy, radiation, and surgery, her oncologist told her that she would prove the statistics wrong.

During her treatment, Lois met many people who expressed their need to share their experiences with others going through the same thing. Out of this need, she formed a support group and established Victory in the Valley, a nonprofit organization to help patients with cancer. The organization now offers comprehensive support, including statewide support groups, lodging for out-of-town patients, transportation, a special program for children with cancer and their siblings and children who have a parent with cancer, and a "Buddy" program for those newly diagnosed with cancer.

Lois continues to do well, with no sign of recurrence. She offers love, support, and a helping hand to those going through the cancer experience. Her life is an example that good things can come from some of life's most difficult journeys. Victory can surface in the valley of cancer.

Diana Thomi, RN
Daughter of 14-year breast cancer survivor
Kansas

I don't borrow from the future. I accept that now is the best time of my life. After my diagnosis of cancer, my life is different, but my change in attitude has made it more rewarding.

Florence Langer
Survivor of breast cancer and recurrence
Ohio

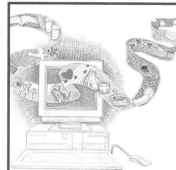

Computer Companions

I attribute part of the success of being cancer free to the positive attitude the Cancer Survivors chat group has given me.

I am in the U.S. Foreign Service. While posted to the U.S. Embassy in New Delhi, India, I developed back pain. The doctor said I had pulled muscles. I took ibuprofen, and life went on as usual. After moving to Sofia, Bulgaria, I started to experience more severe pain that ran down my left leg. I also had fevers and chills. Then I started having night sweats. I finally went to our nurse, who decided to send me to London for tests.

In London, after multiple tests, the doctors found a spot on my lung and a swollen lymph node on my upper left chest. They did a biopsy and discovered that I had Hodgkin's disease. I started talking with doctors at the London Clinic, but the U.S. State Department made me return to the United States for treatment. We had three days to pack our bags!

Once in the United States, tests showed extensive involvement. The picture was bleak. I underwent six cycles of chemotherapy, which lasted six months.

My last chemotherapy was July 28, 1994. After that, tests showed I was in remission! My physician said that since I was at such an advanced stage of disease, I had about a 50% risk of recurrence. He recommended a bone marrow transplant (BMT). I started doing my homework and went to consultations. In my case, since I had not relapsed right away, the odds of long-term remission were approximately the same if I had a BMT now or waited for the first relapse. That, along with the risks of a BMT, made me wait.

As a precaution, though, I had an apheresis for peripheral blood stem cells (my currently good blood cells were stored away)—just in case I need an autologous transplant in the future. Both of my sisters were perfect marrow matches for each other—but not for me.

During my chemotherapy treatment period, I joined the America Online (AOL) computer service. While browsing one day, I found a public chat room called "Cancer Survivors." I went in and found a great group of people held together by two breast cancer survivors.

They had met on-line a few months earlier and started the Cancer Survivors chat room, which met every Monday. I started signing in on Mondays to chat with everyone. We became a tightly knit family. In fact, we grew so much that we reached the limit of the number of people who can be in a chat room. I took it upon myself to ask AOL for a bigger room and more cancer resources. Finally, after some letter-writing campaigns, the company gave us a bigger room in the newly created American Cancer Society area. We were on our way.

Since August 1994, I have been cancer-free. I attribute part of my success to the positive attitude the Cancer Survivors chat group has given me. I have also branched out. I created a popular World Wide Web site on the Internet to help people find information on lymphoma. To me, it is a way of giving back to the community that helped me so much.

Mike Barela
web site: Lymphoma Resource Pages
http://www.alumni.caltech.edu/~mike/lymphoma.html

Visiting with the people in the chemotherapy room can be quite an uplifting and humbling experience. Yes, I cried a few times for some of them. None of us is sure when his or her life clock will expire. We are just more aware that it is a greater possibility from where we now stand in the cancer situation. Cancer is not a death sentence anymore. It's an eye opener and a reflector of where you are in your life. Cancer reminds you of the need to prioritize: God, husband, family, then work. My walk with Jesus Christ is closer. Yes, I still have a lot of questions. Some will never get answered on this side of Heaven—but He's there, He's been there, and He will always be there. He promised.

Carolynn Sue Harrison
Wife, mother, and cancer survivor
Indiana

Where Do Rainbows Go?

Where do rainbows go
Some say they don't know

Do they hide in my garden hose
In a tear on my child's nose
Do they hide in a piece of glass
Or on a blade of summer grass

Where do rainbows go
Do they sit on my window pane
After a soft spring rain
Or do they hide in tall, oaken trees
And in the color of fallen leaves

Where do rainbows go
It is heard that some have said
That rainbows sleep in flower beds
And others say that a rainbow's gold
Is found at the bottom of goldfish bowls

Where do rainbows go
With all I have seen and know
I do know where rainbows go
I think if you use your mind to see
You'll find that rainbows hide in you and me

I was feeling deep despair and wondered where God's promise had gone. I began to write this poem. When my eight-year-old son, Matthew, came home from school, he sat on the couch with me and wanted to read what I had written. As I read the poem, the sun came shining through the window and reflected off my diamond wedding band. We both looked up in amazement as we saw it make a beautiful rainbow that filled the wall beside us! God's promise was so evident!

Elaine Metzung
Mother of three young children and
breast cancer survivor
Ohio

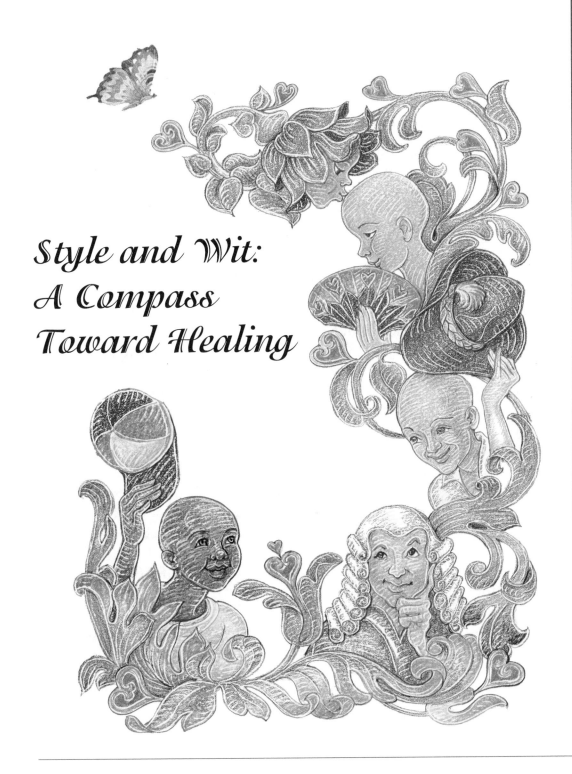

Chapter 5

Style and Wit: A Compass Toward Healing

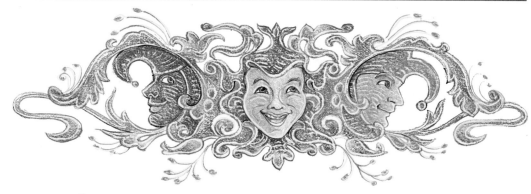

Twelve Steps to Recovery of a Sense of Humor

There is no magic wand to take away the pain of our trials and tribulations; through humor we can hasten the healing.

The bad news is, the chemotherapy made all my hair fall out. The good news is, I am now eligible for *both* leading roles in "The King and I." Laughing over that joke 10 years ago didn't make my life-threatening disease disappear. But, by spotting some humor in my circumstances—some comedy amid the chaos of cancer—I found the strength to get through some tough times. I understood what research had proven: there are psychological and physiological benefits to laughter and humor. Laughter reduces muscle tension, lowers blood pressure, improves blood circulation, deepens breathing, and aids digestion. It releases endorphins, the body's natural pain killers that can relieve stress. Humor increases communication, lowers conflict and anger, increases a sense of well-being, and facilitates learning. It provides distraction—a mental vacation—that allows for a detached viewpoint—a "cosmic perspective." Healing humor (i.e., "laughing with") provides all these benefits. Toxic humor (i.e., "laughing at"), however, does not.

Drawing on my experience as a psychotherapist and a cancer survivor, I have applied the teachings of Norman Cousins, Allen Klein, and others to come up with **Twelve Steps to Recovery of a Sense of Humor.**

1. **Expect the best, but prepare for the worst.** Choose your own personal punch line to have ready for your next crisis. Some favorites are
    • "Are we having fun yet?"
    • "Beam me up, Scotty!"

- "Take it back! It's not what I ordered!"
- "Discover wildlife! Have kids!"
- "I'd rather be (sailing, dancing, skiing)!"
- "I refuse to be intimidated by reality!"
- "Toto, I've a feeling we're not in Kansas anymore!"

2. **Make up a joke about your problem** (e.g., bad news/good news, knock, knock . . .) "The bad news is my suitcase broke into pieces as it came off the plane. The good news is it was the first one off the baggage chute, and the second, and the third . . ." "One writer sent this note in response to yet another publishing rejection: 'I regret to inform you that your rejection notice does not meet my editorial needs.'"

3. **Exaggerate or diminish the problem until it is so absurd, you have to laugh**. "Yes, dinner's late again. Alert the media!" One business woman took her unaccepted budget to the copier, made it the size of a postage stamp, then presented it to her boss as her "reduced budget."

4. **Recall a funny, playful time in your childhood.** Decide what elements made it so. Then, make it a part of your life today. Now imagine yourself at age 100. Looking back on your life, what fun would you regret missing? Then do it now!

5. **Select an affirmation or visualization and say or picture it often**. Mine were "Every day, in every way, I'm getting better and better!" "This is a great opportunity, brilliantly disguised as an impossible situation!" and "Don't sweat the small stuff; it's *all* small stuff." My visualization was picturing myself radiantly healthy, basking on a beach, one year post-bone marrow transplant. Aaahhh!

6. **Practice optimism.** I chose to see 50/50 odds for survival as the cup being half full—a 50% chance was more than without a transplant. Realizing that it could have been worse keeps things in balanced perspective.

7. **Create your unique props or power-laugh reminders.** Consider "Candid Camera" tapes, funny movies, or *I Love Lucy* comedies; displays of zany photos, cartoons, and jokes on mirrors and doors; masks, wigs, hats, costumes, and gadgets; a "Get Out of Jail Free" card to

present to the next traffic officer you encounter; a red clown nose to wear while trying to wake the kids on school days; and inflatable legs or hands to stick out of unexpected places. When my hair began falling out from chemotherapy, I had it shaved into a mohawk as I bade it farewell.

8. **Encourage smiles and laughter.** Place an adhesive dot on your watch to remind you to smile. One man, with facial paralysis and an eye patch, printed "I'm smiling on the inside" on the patch, which made those around him smile even though he could not.

9. **Draw your "demon" or name your "monster" (i.e., whomever or whatever gives you trouble).** My monster was an infusion pump that used to beep at all hours of the night. We named it "R2D2," and a relationship was born. Named computers become user-friendlier. One organization called theirs "Elvis."

10. **Let go.** Write down your worries and burn them or tie them to a helium balloon, then release them or mail them to the North Pole. Caution: Do *not* put your return address on the envelope. I did, and a few days later, all my troubles were returned to me.

11. **Discover the advantage to past disadvantages.** Recall prior setbacks that ultimately were overcome or became beneficial to you. Before first grade, I panicked about whether I'd be able to learn to read; the outcome—I did. Remember how impossible riding a bike felt just before it clicked in? A broken romance, after which you swore you could never love again, but did?

12. **Learn to laugh at yourself.** They say angels can fly because they take themselves lightly.

Potential laughter is all around us. If we just look for it, we will find it, even in the most mundane places. Once, at a laundromat, I noticed a sign that said, "When the machine stops, please remove all your clothing."

Life is a wonderful adventure. However, we must learn to expect, accept, and even embrace the fact that, at times, it isn't logical or fair. There is no magic wand to take away the pain of our trials and tribulations. Through humor, however, we can hasten the healing.

Clare Buie Chaney, PhD
Licensed professional counselor and 10-year leukemia survivor
Texas

The Field Trip

As I awoke that morning to the sound of the cool fall wind, I was disappointed because I had been wishing for a nice day. I teach fourth grade, and my class was taking a field trip to the fire station that day. I had planned ahead by inviting my teacher aide and a parent to go with us on the trip, which was about a seven-block hike. I was taking chemotherapy at the time, so I needed backup resources in case I couldn't go the distance. As I thought about the weather and what clothing was appropriate, I decided I should wear a heavy sweater and slacks. I have a double mastectomy, so I put on my bra and prostheses . . . or so I thought.

The field trip went very well, and we were just about to enter the school door when something possessed me to feel for my prostheses. They weren't there! Sheer panic spread through me. I hurried the students into the school and called my aide over. I told her my "boobs" must have fallen out somewhere along the way. She about died laughing but said she would go back and look for them. Surely they would be nearby.

Well, off she went on her search for the missing boobs. She looked in the street gutters, through the piles of leaves along the way, and any other place she could think of. They were nowhere to be found. As the day wore on, the story about my lost boobs soon became common knowledge among my peers. Each time the story was told, it increased in humor—for me and for them. Some were teasing that they would put it on the local advertising channel that two "boobs" were missing somewhere between Grant Elementary and the firehouse.

When I arrived home that afternoon, I realized what had happened. While struggling with the dilemma about what to wear, I put on my bra but forgot the prostheses. The boobs were safe at home on my dresser.

Darlene Bierwagen
Breast cancer survivor
Wyoming

The Dance Remedy

As long as I hear "good" stories,
I throw off my fears
and believe I'm getting well.

In May of 1994, I was in the hospital for experimental chemotherapy for breast cancer. A week after receiving a high dosage, my white blood cell count dropped to 100 (normal is 5,000–10,000). As a preventive measure, I received powerful antibiotics intravenously and was confined to my room because my immune system was very weak. My visitors scrubbed their hands and donned surgical masks before entering. The white blood cell count edged up slowly over the next two weeks, but my immune system remained greatly compromised.

I had insomnia and tried to rest by listening to classical music on the radio I had brought from home. At 11 pm, the announcer said he was about to play "agitating" music and put on a 16th century tarantella. It had a solid, infectious beat played on wonderful old instruments—nasal reeds and small drums. I was seized with a compulsion to leap from the bed and dance wildly.

Imagine what I must have looked like: a one-breasted 43-year-old woman, completely bald, barefoot, with flowing hospital gowns both front and back. I was attached to a tube snaking from a hole in my chest to the IV pole, which had become my constant companion since coming to the hospital. I was a woman possessed by this music, in the throes of a frenzied jig.

My exertion was exhausting me, but still the music throbbed. I told myself to sit down and catch my breath, but I couldn't seem to stop. When the music finally ended, I collapsed on the bed and listened as the announcer explained the development of the tarantella. There were a lot of spiders (including tarantulas) in Renaissance Italy and no medical antidote to their poison. The superstition held that a bite victim might survive by dancing until he dropped. Therefore, the local musicians were called upon to perform music to promote his activity. "Aha!" I said, gasping on my bed. "The chemotherapy within me must resemble spider venom."

To amuse my morning nurse, I told her of my midnight romp. She replied, "But it's not superstition; it really works. Frenetic activity stimulates the body to release epinephrine, and this natural antihistamine counteracts the allergic reaction to the spider bite." Could the same be said about a reaction to chemotherapy? She shrugged.

Later that same day, she came in to tell me my white counts had jumped from 700 to 3,850!

Quite suddenly, I was no longer neutropenic. Now I was free to roam the halls, and my IV was discontinued and disconnected. Within 24 hours, with normal counts, I was sent home, holding the record for the shortest stay of any woman on that protocol.

Call it the dance remedy.

Carolyn Keiler Paul
Novelist and advanced breast cancer survivor
Massachusetts

Though Mary had a very curable cancer,
we discussed how there was no such thing as
a case of "Cancer Lite"—either physically
or emotionally.

Morry Edwards, PhD
Doctor of Mary, a patient with lymphoma
Michigan

I told my son, "Spencer, I hope every
mosquito that bites me this summer dies
from the chemotherapy!" He quickly
replied, "Either that, Mom, or there are
going to be a lot of bald-headed mosquitos
at Hide-A-Way Lake this summer!"

Dody Stovall
Seven-year breast cancer survivor
Texas

Boxer Boldness

Many of our friends and relatives had been asking if they could help in any way. I decided to take them up on their offers. . . .

Have you noticed all the wild and crazy boxer shorts that are in department stores? Have you ever wondered who would buy them? Have you ever met a guy who had 43 pairs? Meet my husband, Dick Kimberly.

His prostate cancer was diagnosed in February of 1995. He had surgery in March, and the recovery seemed to go on forever. Every aspect of the recovery seemed longer and harder than what we had anticipated. We were both exhausted and discouraged from months of dealing with cancer when we learned that radiation treatments would also be necessary.

The day that Dick went in to be measured and marked for the radiation treatments was a particularly difficult day. Aside from being tired and scared, having people poking around in that area of your body is just plain embarrassing! Knowing this would continue daily for six weeks was difficult for him to deal with. He seemed to have reached an all-time low.

My husband is a very positive person and usually very outgoing and friendly. He likes to joke with people and looks at the bright side of things. Even though he was feeling really down, he mentioned to me that he had stopped at a store and bought three pairs of brightly colored underwear to wear to his radiation treatments. He said he had decided that since he needed to undress in front of all those female strangers every day, he thought that they might as well be embarrassed, too. After laughing about his silly idea, I decided to take it a step further.

Many of our friends and relatives had been asking if they could help in any way. I decided to take them up on their offers. I wrote a letter explaining the situation and asked them to send something colorful, naughty or nice, appropriate or inappropriate, with a 34-inch waist ASAP. I mailed this letter to about 30 people.

Within a week, manila envelopes with silly boxer shorts started arriving daily. Dick received Halloween underwear, hot pepper sauce underwear, red satin underwear, dancing pigs underwear, Statue of Liberty underwear—you name it, he got it!

Every day for weeks, we rushed out to check the mail and loved opening the packages, all of which came with notes wishing us well. They brought us the support we needed, some really unusual shorts, and many much-needed laughs.

Therese Foy Kimberly
Wife of prostate cancer survivor
Missouri

One windy day, I was pumping gas into my car. Suddenly, I felt my wig lift off my head and blow away. All of the gas station attendants ran out with their mouths hanging open as I chased my wig and put it back on my bald head. We all had a good laugh. Now when I drive in and they come out to greet me, I tell them that there is a cover charge for the show.

Jeanie Gigliotti
Stage III ovarian cancer survivor
California

One-Day-at-a-Time Attitude

She continues to amaze me and teach me about life.

My mother was first diagnosed with ovarian cancer five years ago. All of us had so many adjustments to make with this diagnosis. My mother has always been there for me as a teacher and role model. She continues to teach me by her example of strength and her "one-day-at-a-time" attitude.

One of the difficult adjustments was the loss of her hair during her chemotherapy treatments. My sisters and I went wig shopping with her to offer her our love and support. This role reversal coupled with her loss of hair seemed to hamper her usual positive spirit. As the weeks and months passed, she seemed to grow ever so slightly more comfortable with the idea of a head with no hair. In fact, she would occasionally walk around the house without the wig when we were visiting. One day, she even forgot about it long enough to go outside to take out the trash without anything on her head. My son, 14 years old at the time, was in her driveway playing basketball. He smiled as he looked up at her and said, "Grandma, I love your Michael Jordan look." This was a turning point for her. Nothing ever seemed quite so bad after that. The hair has since grown back, and Mom continues with her "one-day-at-a-time" attitude. Most of all, she continues to amaze me and teach me about life.

Carol Santalucia
Daughter of an ovarian cancer survivor
Ohio

I Flipped My Wig!

"Comedy is simply a funny way of being serious." —Peter Ustinov

During the summer, I was receiving chemotherapy for my breast cancer. My parents invited me and my three-year-old daughter Sarah to go fishing and camping with them. I wore a wig to protect my hairless head and a sun visor to protect my face from the sun while we fished from the boat. Sarah squealed with delight each time her grandma had a bite and pulled her line in. Her eagerness was so contagious that even I became excited at the anticipation of catching a fish.

On one particular cast, Grandma thought she had a catch. Sarah was all eyes waiting for her to bring that fish into the boat. My mother soon realized it wasn't a fish but rather a stick caught on her line. She announced with fake excitement, "I caught a stick fish!" My daughter became very excited, stood up, and started shouting, "Grandma caught a stick fish! Grandma caught a stick fish! Can I see it Grandma?" We all started laughing at Sarah's pure, childlike enthusiasm and enjoyment over the "stick fish."

It was a warm day but the sun had gone behind the clouds, so I took off my sun visor. In the process of doing so, my wig got caught in it. As I pulled the visor, my wig flew up into the air and came back down into the boat. It landed directly over the worm can on the seat next to me, just as if it were a wig stand. Roaring with laughter, I announced, "That was so funny that I flipped my wig!"

It made for a humorous story to tell my husband, aunt, and uncle around the campfire that night. I still chuckle to myself whenever I remember the day I flipped my wig.

Kathleen Schoendorf, RN
Thirteen-year breast cancer survivor,
American Cancer Society volunteer, and nurse
Wisconsin

The Affair

Humorous images never fail to help me put the problematic and painful in perspective and regain my composure in public. When anger and pain mount, one gentle nudge from humor restores balance. In a very profound way, humor makes life worth living.

Humor is a vital weapon in the arsenal aimed at managing stress. A quick change of pace or a flash of humor can bring instant relief from unbearable pressure. Humor can enhance the ability to function on a more efficient level. A woman in my chemotherapy group helped me, and everyone else, cope with the tremendously stressful situation of the first day of each chemotherapy cycle by sharing a humorous fantasy.

On a Monday, during her second year of treatment, she came running in for her first shot of a new cycle of chemotherapy. She said she had stayed away until the last possible minute so that she could be the last patient and would not have to endure the long wait. After the extensive preliminaries, she took her seat in the hall with the other patients waiting for their treatments. As we all complained about the excessive fatigue we were feeling, she interjected, "I think I'm just too tired to have an affair today." She said it to no one in particular, but the remark drew gales of laughter and a few gasps. "Besides," she continued, "If I had an affair, it would have to be with my doctor, because he is used to one-breasted wonders." All of us were convulsed with laughter. I guess each of us had this thought at one time or another and had sensibly rejected it! We were delighted—and united—in the shared comfort of an outrageous fantasy.

Humor also helps initiate control when events erode balance and threaten to diminish dignity. When I feel I might embarrass myself by bursting suddenly into uncontrollable tears, I evoke an image that I know will make me laugh. Humorous images never fail to help me put the problematic and the painful in perspective and regain my composure in public. When anger and pain mount, one gentle nudge from humor restores balance. In a very profound way, humor makes life worth living.

Rena J. Blumberg
Breast cancer survivor
Ohio

My Knight in Shining Armor

He had a way of making me feel pretty—even with my scars and purple paint. I will always remember him for this special gift.

I was diagnosed with breast cancer at age 30. I underwent a lumpectomy and lymph node dissection. Since my mother died of breast cancer, I wanted to do everything in my power to defeat mine. I chose to undergo both chemotherapy and radiation treatments.

When I went to my first radiation treatment, I was pleasantly surprised to find that my doctor resembled the movie star Harrison Ford. He was really a wonderful care provider, and not only because he resembled Harrison Ford. He was very kind and gentle. Surprisingly, this made the radiation treatments a little more bearable, and I looked forward to these visits. Amazingly, my libido was still alive—even in the midst of breast cancer treatment. You know how some women "fall in love" with their obstetricians? Well . . .

During my first visit, the radiation therapy assistants took very precise measurements and x-rays of my right breast and underarm. They marked the measurements on my skin in purple ink, which would be my "war paint" for the next eight weeks. I looked like the bionic woman. I went to radiation therapy five times a week. I had to lie on my back on a cold table while an enormous machine was positioned directly above my breast area.

During my final radiation treatments, I was placed under a different radiation machine where I had to remain very still. The machine had to be lowered right down to the scar on my breast. My doctor stood at the end of the table with his hands lightly on my head. He leaned down and whispered three magical words: "I'll protect you." Talk about great medicine! I was on Cloud Nine for the next few days! He had a way of making me feel pretty even with my scars and purple paint. I will always remember him for this special gift.

Linda Scheele
Eight-year survivor of breast cancer
Washington

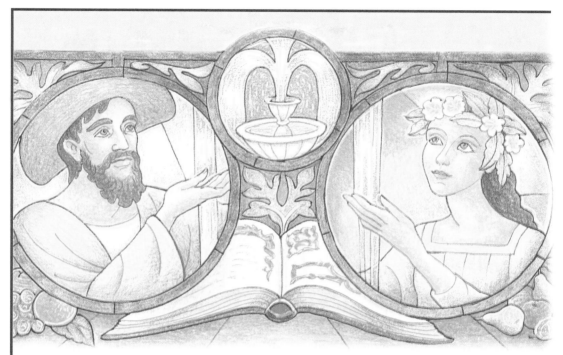

Knowledge Is Both Powerful and Humorous

I read everything I could get my hands on.
If knowledge is power, I wanted to be omniscient!

In 1995, I was diagnosed with inflammatory breast cancer. Once the initial shock wore off a little, the first rounds of tears were dried, and every test known to mankind was run, I began a treatment regimen and was on the road to recovery.

During the next eight months, I received four chemotherapy treatments, four surgeries (including the removal of my left breast), a stem-cell transplant, and radiation therapy. Throughout all of this, I became an avid reader. I read about every drug, every pill, and every treatment prescribed—especially the side effects. Yes, I read everything I could get my hands on. If knowledge is power, I wanted to be omniscient! Anything I didn't quite understand, I would ask about. One afternoon, I called the doctor's office to ask what "feelings of impending death" felt like so I could tell if I was experiencing that side effect or not.

One day, as I was reading a nutritional healing reference book, which also described different kinds of cancers and some beneficial foods, I realized my coffee cup was nearly empty. So, I went to the stove for a refill. Unbeknownst to me, a page or two flipped in the book while I was refilling my coffee. As I continued to read, I was not aware that I had skipped several pages. As I read further, I realized there were several symptoms I had not experienced—not yet anyway. The more I read, the more concerned I became.

By the time my husband arrived home from his job in retail sales, I was at least one bubble off plumb—one taco short of a full combination plate—my dipstick was not touching my oil—just a wee bit left of center—to say the least! He asked, "What's the matter?" I tearfully replied, "I have this . . ." pointing to the paragraph I had been reading. Very calmly he said, "No, you don't." I quickly blurted out, "Oh, yes I do!" After all, I was so knowledgeable from all my reading. Very patiently, he again replied, "No, you don't." With that, I shouted out, "What makes you such an expert? I know that I have this!" Less patient this time, he again replied, "No, you do not have this!" Very sarcastically, I asked, "How can you be so sure?" As he slowly pointed to the page heading "Prostate Cancer," he smiled and emphatically replied, "Because you don't have one!"

Cindy Schwerin
Sixteen-month breast cancer survivor
Colorado

I explain that my lack of memory when I am on chemotherapy is caused by a "chemo-lobotomy."

Carol Kaloger
Four-year ovarian cancer survivor
Florida

To celebrate the end of chemo, I had a "no mo' chemo" party. Instead of burning my bra, I burned all my wigs and scarfs. I can't wait to get my hair back. There's no way I'll ever have a bad hair day!

Dody Stovall
Seven-year breast cancer survivor
Texas

Not by Choice

She disliked having people stare at her bald head, so she created a line of T-shirts, sweatshirts, and caps to help others deal humorously with the problem.

How can any family survive having two children be afflicted with rare cancerous tumors? The Christianson family found that a sense of humor and faith in God made all the difference in helping them defeat cancer and counter the stigma associated with the illness.

Kristen Christianson and her brother Scott are both cancer survivors. Scott was 18 years old when he was diagnosed with a rare form of cancer called African Burkitt's lymphoma. Kris was 17 when diagnosed with an equally rare form of cancer called spindle cell sarcoma. Both were treated successfully at the University of Wisconsin Comprehensive Cancer Center. Scott has been in remission for more than 12 years, and Kris has been disease-free for more than 8 years. Both have an excellent prognosis.

While undergoing aggressive chemotherapy, they, like many others, suffered unpleasant side effects, including hair loss. Scott dealt with the problem by donning a wig with long, red curls as a joke or wearing a cap. Kris usually opted for bandanas. However, she disliked having people stare at her bald head, so she created a line of T-shirts, sweatshirts, and caps to help others deal humorously with the problem.

The items include the phrase "Hair by Chemo" on the front and feature an illustration of a scissors and comb inside the international circle-and-slash symbol for "no." On the back is the phrase "Not by Choice." The logo helps people hold their heads high and puts a smile of understanding on the faces of curious onlookers.

Today, while Scott and Kris pursue new lives, their mother has taken over the business. The enterprise is not financially "successful." Rather, Mrs. Christianson's reward comes from giving people ideas of how to cope, especially during the stressful first year out, when fear of recurrence is at its height. She shares with others how a sense of humor and trust in God made their family stronger.

Helen Whitman-Obert, HHW, RN, CNM
Nurse manager on the oncology unit where both Scott and Kris were treated
Wisconsin

Double-Checked

Though gripped with apprehension, he had a bedrock confidence in his Lord, Jesus Christ, to carry him through whatever lay ahead.

The honeycomb of white lights over the operating table dazzled the young man as he felt multiple pairs of hands guiding him from the stretcher. The table seemed too narrow to hold him despite the fact that he was gaunt from months of vomiting nearly everything he ate. The calm, professional voices swirled around him, but his heart pounded louder than the words they were saying. He felt so cold that his fingers and toes hurt. He knew that many friends were praying earnestly for him and that his family, 1,500 miles away in another country, was also praying, yet none of these people were in the room with him. He was surrounded by unfamiliar faces, half-hidden behind masks, speaking in medical terms he could not comprehend. He was most grateful at this moment for the presence of the God to whom he trusted his life. Though gripped with apprehension, he had a bedrock confidence in his Lord, Jesus Christ, to carry him through whatever lay ahead.

The doctors had agreed that it was most certainly a malignancy. This opinion was based on the various biopsies they had taken by means of a scope put through the young man's mouth and into his stomach. What kind of cancer it was, however, remained uncertain; thus, he had consented to having his stomach cut open and examined directly. Here, today, it was happening. The result might determine the future of his graduate education, the hopes for a ministry back in his native land, all that he had sacrificed so much for.

The pace picked up in the operating room. The voices spoke more quickly; figures moved in practiced routine. Nothing about it was routine for the young man, and he understood little of what he saw and heard, except the information that the surgeon was "scrubbing" outside of the room. Suddenly, hands lifted the hospital gown up and away from the man's stomach and chest as someone explained that electrodes for a heart monitor had to be placed on his chest.

Then they all stopped—first the one lifting his gown, then each of the other figures in the room. Moving closer to the table, they peered at the bright yellow circle already sticking to the patient's skin, just under his left ribs and directly over the spot where the surgeon planned to cut. The sticker bore the familiar arches of the McDonald's restaurant logo, and emblazoned across it were the words "Double-Checked for Accuracy." Two red check marks pierced the words.

He couldn't see behind their masks, but he knew they were smiling. Chuckles broke through the serious atmosphere. One staff member walked to the door to call the surgeon in from the scrub sink to look at the sticker, which had originally resided on the wrapping of a special-order burger. The young man and his friends had eaten these burgers on their way home from the doctor's office after he had made the decision for surgery.

As the laughter subsided, the surgeon assured the young man that he would indeed double-check his work and that accuracy held a high priority. The young man's tension seemed to dissipate into the laughter all around him. Now he didn't even mind the sting of the IV medicine as the mask came down over his face. Breathe deeply . . . and have a good laugh.

Pamela Popovich, RN, BS, OCN®
Oncology nurse and friend of survivor
Illinois

My friend said she was prepared to lose her hair, but losing her eyebrows was a shock. She never got the hang of painting them on. Every morning she went to work with "celebrity" eyebrows. One eyebrow looked like Jean Harlow, and the other looked like Gene Shalit.

Cindy H. Melancon
Five-year ovarian cancer survivor and thriver, celebrating life today!
Texas

"What About Wet T-Shirt Contests?"

It's because they support me with humor—and love me for who I am, not what I look like—that makes me laugh and cry at the same time.

"*Breast* cancer? Can't it be some other body part, please? Why not . . . butt cancer?!" I could use a butt-ectomy. But hey, half my wardrobe depends on a perky set of tits! We're talking big investment here— dozens of skimpy halter tops emblazoned with logos like "Hot Sex." However, when word about my diagnosis got out to my biker friends, they were unsympathetic about the wardrobe thing. Their advice: "Fight! Get rid of the thing. Boobs are fun, but 'live to ride!'"

After my surgery for breast cancer, I heard many varied responses from my biker friends. One fellow contemplated my chest and stated that he had a great plan for the perfect Halloween costume. I could dress half and half—a woman on one side, and a *man* on the other side! It's an idea. My girlfriend panicked: "What about wet T-shirt contests?" The general consensus was that I should go ahead and enter. What could happen? They might toss only half the money that they did before—or maybe twice as much for the novelty value? (Bet you didn't know wet T-shirt contests were charity events. Why else, hmmm?)

There also were sly references to one-eyed pirate-types needing only one boob to gawk at. Other dumb stuff like that makes me laugh. It's because they support me with humor—and love me for who I am, not what I look like—that makes me laugh and cry at the same time. I love them back, twice as much as before, and hopefully for a long time.

Sandy Purser-Carlsten
Five-year breast cancer survivor
California

Just Following the Doctor's Orders!

My father-in-law is a dairy farmer. After years of working outdoors in the harsh sun and tending the fields and animals, he developed skin cancer on his face. He periodically needed to have skin lesions removed at his local physician's office. During each visit, his doctor reminded him to use sun block on his face and exposed skin and, whenever possible, limit his amount of sun exposure. This advice is easier said than done for a farmer.

Dad loves farming and being his own boss. By nature, he hates attending to details, or, as he calls it, "fine work." He also routinely forgets to apply sun block upon leaving the house in the morning and cannot be bothered to return home just for that detail. Recently, his physician told him that he needed to pay closer attention to applying sun block daily. To encourage better compliance with the doctor's orders, my mother-in-law put a handy pump dispenser in the bathroom so Dad would not forget to apply the lotion each morning.

After about a week of daily use, my father-in-law became worried because his face and hands were increasingly dry and itchy. The long hours driving the tractor in the sunlight apparently were wreaking havoc on his exposed skin in a new way, even with the use of sun block. How could this happen when he finally was applying the lotion faithfully? This would require another trip to the physician, although the appointment would have to wait until next week when Dad could take a break from his field work.

Unlike my father-in-law, my mother-in-law's nature is to attend to the details and "fine work." While cleaning their bathroom, she noticed that the soap dispenser was nearly empty after filling it only a week ago. With a little investigation, she determined that Dad had been applying liquid soap to his face and hands from the old soap dispenser, which was near the dispenser containing the sun block. Thus, Mom was able to eliminate Dad's mysterious symptoms and the need for another visit to the doctor.

James G. Wollet
Son-in-law of skin cancer survivor
Wisconsin

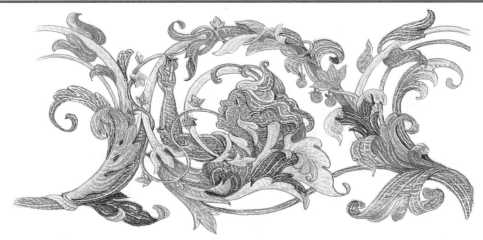

Being a "First"

Lisa was 17 years old when she was diagnosed with a liver tumor. Upon realizing that her hair would fall out following her chemotherapy treatments, this spirited young lady decided to dye her hair purple!

Lisa was one of the first patients with cancer at Cleveland Clinic to receive a liver transplant. Typical of Lisa, she did very well. Later, while on cyclosporin (an antirejection drug), Lisa became pregnant. She refused the option of having an abortion. Lisa went on to become one of the first patients in the area to carry a baby to full term while on cyclosporin. She delivered a healthy, normal baby boy! A lot of firsts for one courageous lady!

Ann Birkmire, RN, MSN
Pediatric clinical nurse specialist
Massachusetts

Halloween marked the one-year
anniversary of my first chemotherapy
treatment. I like to think of it as having
chased the goblins away.

Patricia L. Kinney
Breast cancer and bone marrow transplant
survivor, a.k.a. "Alive and well!"
Arizona

The Green Glow

As a team, patients, their families, and nurses can turn a crisis into an opportunity, turn tears into laughter, build bridges beyond the walls, and use humor to keep the glow alive.

As an oncology nurse, I remind patients and families of the potential for hair loss as a side effect of chemotherapy. I also quickly add that this is temporary, and hair will grow back when the treatments are completed. To provide support to my patient "Joe" and his wife, I answered his questions and explained that hair loss usually begins about a week after treatment. Joe quietly answered, "Yes . . . I know." Immediately, his wife stated, "He has already had 'The Green Glow.'" I was surprised by the intensity and seriousness in her voice. The clinic nurse looked at me, puzzled, as if to ask, "Why didn't you tell me about that side effect?" Joe's wife continued, "Yes . . . 'The Green Glow,' it happened last night. Show her." I was becoming both puzzled and curious. During my past 16 years as an oncology nurse, I have never heard of any green glow. Suddenly, Joe began to laugh uncontrollably. After he finally regained his composure, Joe explained, "I went to M.J. Designs yesterday and bought some of that green hair color that glows in the dark. I put it on and showed my wife when she came home from work." In the meantime, Joe's wife was sitting in absolute silence. Finally, the silence was broken as she quietly asked, "You mean it wasn't a side effect? You mean it wasn't the chemotherapy?" Now we were all laughing, including Joe and his wife.

I couldn't resist carrying the joke one step further. I asked, "When do you start radiation treatments?" Joe replied, "Tomorrow. I will have to come 10 times." This potential for a joke was too much for all of us to pass up. Joe agreed to bring in "The Green Glow" on his last treatment, and his wife would page me when he arrived. I then would take him to the radiation oncologist to see this "new" side effect of radiation. We all eagerly awaited that last treatment. All of us left the clinic that day laughing.

Later that evening, during our cancer support group meeting, the members were sharing stories about how they learned to cope with the crisis of hair loss from chemotherapy. I shared the "green glow" story with them. After the group ended, the husband of one of the patients stopped to thank me for sharing the story. He added, with a grin, "I thought you were going to say that the patient dropped his pants." I looked at him with bewilderment. He continued by telling me, "'Green Glow' is a brand of condom."

As a team, patients, their families, and nurses can turn a crisis into an opportunity, turn tears into laughter, build bridges beyond the walls, and use humor to keep the glow alive.

Becky O'Shea, MS, RN, OCN®
Clinical nurse specialist and consultant,
O'Shea Can You See Consulting
Texas

A little "green" humor: I was given a beautiful plant by a friend while I was in the hospital. After I got it home, I carefully watered and tended to it—only to discover eight months later that it was artificial!

Karen Brown-Greenfield
Four-year survivor of ovarian cancer
Florida

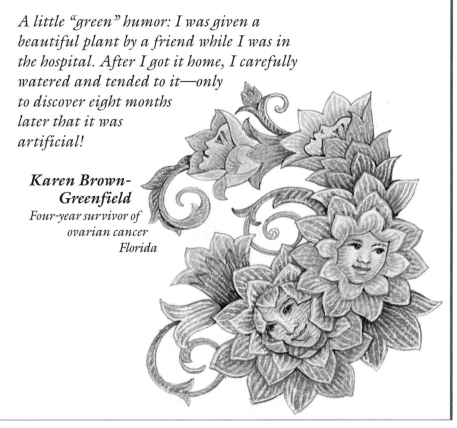

New Doors

I find life very exciting, meaningful, full of hope, and funny.
Laughter airs my soul. I use it every opportunity that I find.

Strange as it may sound, my experience with cancer has revealed many blessings to me. God has watched over me with gentle and loving care as new discovery doors opened for me—doors that I didn't even know existed. The door of journal-keeping has helped me sort out my feelings, hopes, and frustrations. Through the door of self-discovery, I have emerged with a deeper level of comprehension about myself and others. This new understanding has changed my priorities and helped me redefine what is important to me. Always present is my emotional door, which offers me a firm foundation of courage to explore new ideas, hopes, and dreams.

If my cancer had not appeared, I would not have discovered my new, and now cherished, friends. They have profoundly touched my life. I openly share my crazy thoughts, longings, and outrageous ideas. I delight in the healing laughter we share. Through another door, I have discovered how effectively humor frees the moment to make things bearable and lighten my load. Laughter airs my soul. I use it freely with every opportunity that I find.

To help others embrace life, I like to bring sunshine and laughter with a gift of humor. I have the courage and spirit to do the unusual, such as putting on a clown costume for my appointment with the oncologist

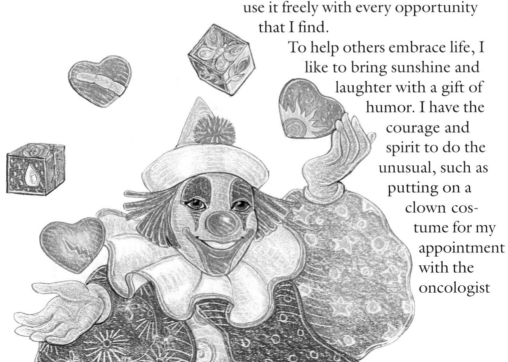

on Halloween. I especially like giving little Snickers® candy bars to complete strangers. I love their reaction—it is so pure and honest. If you have never done this, do it and watch their response. At first they are surprised, which is followed by a heartfelt thanks that a stranger would give them a gift. If I can bring a smile to a face or brighten someone's life with a Snickers, think of all the loving opportunities that await you and me through the simple giving of ourselves.

I gladly open my doors and let life sweep in. Now, I take the time to feel within, to listen within, and to respond from within. I am grateful for these new doors, which have blessed me with so many opportunities to give and receive gifts of joy, inspiration, encouragement, and creativity. I find life very exciting, meaningful, full of hope, and funny. I wonder, would I have found this if I had not gone through my cancer experience?

Patti Lewis
Writer, liturgical designer, clergy spouse,
and two-year breast cancer survivor
Arizona

After 48 years of eating practically anything, it's not easy to give up some of your favorite foods or the way they are prepared. But, the thought of dying is harder to take!

(Helen) Paulette Pyles
Young grandmother and 30-month breast cancer survivor
Ohio

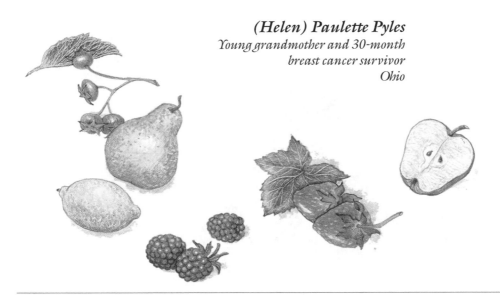

Move Over, Energizer Bunny

With the power of positive thinking, I borrowed the drumsticks of the "Energizer Bunny" so I, too, can keep on going, and going, and going . . .

No amount of cursing or praying would make the grinding engine start. It really didn't matter, though, because I had no energy to curse or pray anyway. I dragged myself back into the house and called my dad for a ride. "Dad, I need a ride to the doctor's office to get my blood-work done," I told him.

He promptly answered, "I'll be there in a minute." Once again, Dad came to my rescue. When he arrived, I sprang from the door to prevent his usual ritual of lifting the hood and fiddling with the engine while expressing his profound knowledge of car mechanics. Reading his mind, I quickly said, "Yes, Dad, we will get a battery when the barbaric blood task is finished."

The battery store yard was filled with farm trucks. I told Dad that I did not want to go in. I was in no mood to listen to crop reports, updates on grandchildren, and who had died. As the door swung open, Dad came out grinning and carrying a battery that he stated was a "real deal." It was difficult to stifle my laughter as Dad jumped into the truck—the new battery had a greater life expectancy than I had! Does chemotherapy have a strange effect on one's sense of humor?

With the power of positive thinking, I borrowed the drumsticks of the "Energizer Bunny" so I, too, can keep on going, and going, and going. . . .

Deborah Wade
Breast cancer survivor
North Carolina

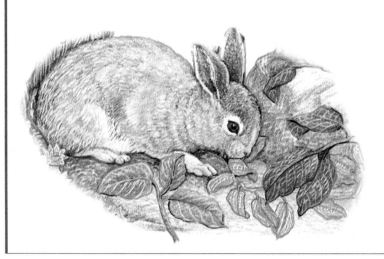

Feeling Lucky

I was feeling lucky despite a diagnosis of pancreatic cancer and surgery that was not successful in removing the tumor. I wanted a SuperLotto ticket! Since my various tubes, IVs, and other entanglements had been removed that morning, I quietly made my way out a side door at the Cleveland Clinic and walked down Euclid Avenue to a store that sold lottery tickets. My healing abdominal incision did slow me down a bit, and my medical student was horrified upon my return—but I did catch a smile on the corner of her mouth.

My ticket was not a winning one, but it did feel delicious to go AWOL and do what I damn well wanted to do.

Now, six years later, after radiation, chemotherapy, and a second surgery, I still buy lottery tickets, and they are never winners. Instead of going AWOL from the hospital, these days I refuse any more CT scans, and I still see a smile on the corner of my doctor's mouth. And it still feels delicious to be a bad boy!

Peter B. Halbin
Writer and cancer survivor who volunteers as a
friendly visitor with newly diagnosed
patients with cancer and their families
Ohio

Finding Joy in All Circumstances

Having cancer reset my priorities. My family and I cherish every moment together. We thank the Lord for this experience because we learned how to find joy in all circumstances.

My family and I found joy and laughter in the midst of my being diagnosed and treated for breast cancer. I'd like to share some of the funny experiences that we had during my surgery, chemotherapy, bone marrow transplant, radiation therapy, and recovery period. They still bring laughter to me every time I share them with others.

My hair began to fall out after I started receiving chemotherapy treatments. I asked my husband to shave it all off rather than have it slowly drift away. Reluctantly, he did so, and our new household motto became "Bald is beautiful!" My young children had a blast drawing tattoos on my bald head with washable markers. We also saved a lock of my hair in a jar. We wrote down what color we each thought it would be when it grew back. None of us guessed that my previously straight, light-brown hair would return as dark brown and curly. It is so curly that I no longer need to get a permanent. During my time without hair (about nine months), I was haircut-free, shampoo-less, and hassle-free. It only took me five minutes to get ready to go out. At home, I either wore turbans or enjoyed the freedom of no hair. I always kept my wig by the front door just in case an unexpected visitor arrived. On several occasions, I simply forgot I was bald; wigless, I once encountered a surprised Culligan man, and I also had some other funny incidents, such as putting it on in a hurry . . . backwards or sideways.

The best benefit of the cancer experience was the new friends I made and all the love, prayers, and joy that was poured out to me by others during my treatment. I am 37, and it has been almost two years since my diagnosis. I am finally back to myself again. Having cancer reset my priorities. My family and I are happy and healthy. We cherish each moment we share together. We thank the Lord for this experience because we learned how to find joy in all circumstances.

Ann Z. Chan
Oncologist's wife with breast cancer
Michigan

Coping With Southern Style

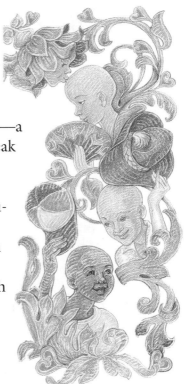

Mrs. Lane was a delightful, elderly lady, and a lady in every sense of the word. She had a passion for hats and for the Kentucky Derby. Her business—a consignment shop—fit her regal, independent streak perfectly. On her first hospitalization, she clearly stated, "I never let stress bother me." She was diagnosed with non-Hodgkin's lymphoma in January and proceeded with her outpatient chemotherapy treatments through the spring. A problem she encountered was that all her friends would repeatedly ask her what was wrong with her. Enough was enough, and in a very Southern fashion, she had calling cards designed to hand to all her friends and colleagues, declaring her stand on the cancer issue:

Announcing
Foy Lane is the proud,
albeit somewhat reluctant, host of
Diffuse Histocytic Non-Hodgkin's Lymphoma.
Since this guest came unannounced, she intends to
be as inhospitable as possible in hopes that it
will not stick around too long.

Mrs. Lane did not let her "guest" rob her of her love for life. Her card remains in my office as a symbol of how hope and humor can be used to face life's adversities the same way one lives life each day.

Sharon Gentry, RN, BSN, OCN®
Oncology case manager
North Carolina

Holder of the Golden Bucket

Since this was an Olympic year, I saw how this simple gesture of love and caring is an art and sports event all its own.

Chemotherapy often has a bad side effect—vomiting. Sometimes, patients are not in the condition to help themselves. As care providers, we lovingly come to their aid. During the 1996 Olympic year, I reflected on this simple gesture of love and caring as an art and sports event all its own.

How many of us have left our loved ones in a different room following chemotherapy to allow him or her an opportunity to rest and recover? We fine-tune our hearing to listen for any signs of need. Hearing my wife call out, "Honey, bring the bucket!" triggers a response in me similar to the starter's pistol for an Olympic runner. I leap out of the chair and dash through the four rooms that lie between me and my finish line. Avoiding the furniture, careening around the corners, nearly falling as I hit the kitchen linoleum in my socks, I reach the bedroom in time to snatch the bucket and place it under my wife's chin. Although I never have timed it, I swear I have lopped off precious seconds to beat my wife's physiological clock each time the call was made.

Now the "art" of holding the bucket comes into play. Will this event be a drool or a full blow-out? If I hold the bucket too far away from her and she drools, then I have missed the target and I am automatically entered into the laundry event. If I don't observe her body language and hold the bucket close to her when, in fact, it should be held at a distance, then I am disqualified from the dash—it didn't even pay to get to her. The bucket holder, a true athlete, needs expert hand-to-eye coordination and quick reflexes to avoid a disaster.

Although we probably have not considered it before, holding the bucket requires great athletic prowess. Some Olympic terms, such as hurling and throwing (up), are applicable. It takes just as much intestinal fortitude to hold the bucket during our event as it does to ski down a mountain, walk the balance beam, or run the marathon.

So, to all the bucket holders out there, hold your buckets high—or low. You are willingly assisting your loved one. It is not a pleasant task, it is not a simple one, but it is one we do gladly without complaint. Consider yourself to be the Golden Bucket Holder in your household. I doubt you will encounter many challengers that have the speed, dexterity, gracefulness, and caring that you do. Now, shine those buckets up and prepare for the next "event."

Richard Vieritz
Husband of a three-year ovarian cancer survivor
Ohio

Humor was the best medicine for me as I moved through cancer. The doctors now recognize my humor as part of my healing process.

Sally Wilson
Survivor of lung cancer with metastasis
Missouri

TAXOL®: A CPA who taxes everything— even cancer!
CISPLATINUM: (Sis Plantin) She plants healing seeds into our bodies.
CYTOXAN®: (Cy Toxin) He sends poison to all cancer cells into our bodies.

Wally Duells
Husband of Kathy, ovarian cancer survivor
Illinois

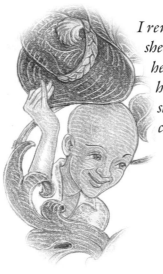

I remember one classmate's confession that she used to look at me and think to herself, "I'm glad I don't have her hairdresser." Of course, that was before she knew that I was getting chemotherapy!

Joanne Hindle, RN, BSN, OCN®
Cancer survivor, oncology nurse, and daughter of cancer survivor
Colorado

Every year Sarah buys a tie for the oncologist who managed her case. The tie includes a little poem:
Another tie,
for another year
that I did not die.

Shay Jacobson, RN, MA
Oncology nurse
Connecticut

Laughter: the antidote for all ills. Good for the mind and soul. I could not have survived without it!

Sally Wilson
Survivor of lung cancer with metastasis
Missouri

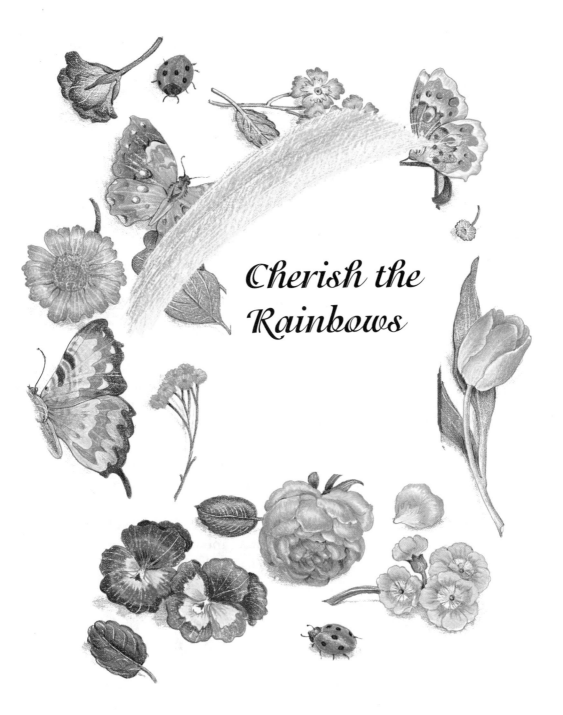

Chapter 6

Cherish the
Rainbows

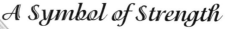

A Symbol of Strength

Sometimes we get so wrapped up in the challenges and struggles of cancer that we forget the strengths that dwell within us. We can all respond to symbols as reminders, even healers, of what we can do, our hopes, courage, and strength.

We inevitably experience moments of despair when our courage fails us. There are times when we have grown weary and days when cancer seems to dominate our lives. Especially during these trying times, symbols serve as tangible reminders of the strength that dwells within us. Many symbols have graced my life during these past five years as I have faced the multiple challenges intrinsic in metastatic breast cancer and several recurrences. However, I must say that I am healthy, my life is rich, and I am blessed. I am a cancer survivor. Symbols of healing have helped me keep the awesomeness and fearfulness of this experience in perspective.

Symbols are personal and unique. They are reminders of what we can strive and hope for. They refortify our courage and strengths. These are a few of the symbols that helped me during my healing process.

A PINK RIBBON PIN for breast cancer awareness, given by a fellow traveler on this journey, symbolizes that we are not alone.

A CLOWN signifies how life-enhancing humor and laughter are to the spirit. He reminds me of many past and present moments of sheer, frivolous, giddy joy.

A LION, small in size, but huge in courage, reminds me of power and control. This symbol was given to me at a time when I was struggling with severe pain. I felt empowered and learned self-hypnosis to deal with the pain. It helped me gain the sense of control that we all need as we face the uncertainty of this unpredictable disease.

An ANGEL was given to me when I was in the throes of deciding whether to pursue a bone marrow transplant. She maintained my focus on hope and strengthened my confidence in a higher power watching over me. I wear a tiny ANGEL PIN on my shoulder every day. She is getting a bit tarnished now, but she is still hanging in there with me.

A GARGOYLE figure was given for luck before my first bone marrow biopsy to symbolize that sometimes we all need a big dose of luck to get us through this journey. A tiny PYRAMID represents the strong base of support that is essential to my healing. It is made of malachite, a stone of transformation, which is ongoing in my life.

A COLLAGE of photographs created before my bone marrow transplant shows my loving family, fun times, kind gestures, and shared moments. This collage was such a vivid reminder of love, support, and caring, as well as a reason to continue.

A copper, Tibetan SINGING BOWL reminds me of the Tibetan monks who go out each day with an empty begging bowl and accept whatever they are given. The bowl prompts me to take one day at a time. What fills my singing bowl is sufficient for today. This alone is cause for singing!

These symbols have been especially meaningful and profound throughout my recovery. Sometimes we get so wrapped up in the challenges and struggles of cancer that we forget the strengths that dwell within us. Symbols are concrete reminders of what is possible. I hope that symbols of love and strength abound in others' lives as well.

Karen Paulsen Brand
Cancer survivor
Minnesota

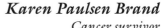

A spotlight has turned on in my life. I see my existence and all the world around me with a deeper sense of awe. The uniqueness that makes us who we are unfolds in an unexpected way when the diagnosis of cancer is made. You discover strength of self, depth of faith, and a desire to stay well that is not matched by any other experience.

Dolores Cornejo, LCSW
Breast cancer survivor and
pediatric oncology social worker
California

A Positive Pansy

I was also blossoming into a whimsical,
lighthearted, courageous creature.

A sign on the door read "Breast Cancer Support Group." The very words jangled my nerves and made my knees knock. I entered the room like a shrinking violet. Two oncology nurses and a social worker greeted me. A caring voice said, "Welcome, we are so glad you are here." I answered shyly, "I would have been here sooner, but I've been recovering from the shingles." Not mentioning the words "breast cancer" suited me very well. The charming ladies in the group gave understanding smiles.

Moments later, another breast cancer survivor slipped into the room. With a hug, we became sisters. For several months, we were the only members of this unique sorority. I saw my new sister gaining strength, showing confidence, and becoming more beautiful both inside and outside. I was also blossoming into a whimsical, lighthearted, courageous creature.

With each meeting, the group began to grow. We now have more than 65 members. As our numbers increased, our philosophy slowly evolved. We selected the name "The Positive Ones." Each time we meet, a speaker shares a bit of professional knowledge. In turn, we share what we have learned with our community of survivors. We share inspirational stories of courage. There truly is power in numbers, and we can see that we are making positive changes in breast cancer care.

Recently, at a support group dinner, I determined that it was the proper time for me to say goodbye. With all the courage I could muster, I stood and said, "I came to this group as a shy, shrinking violet. Thanks to God, my family, and all of you, I leave as a fully grown Positive Pansy. I will miss you. Breast cancer survivors are the happiest people I know. May God bless each one of you."

Norma Anderson Hanna
Four-year breast cancer survivor and
daughter of 13-year breast cancer survivor
Mississippi

Lessons in Life

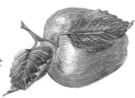

"Stubborn is good. . . . If something does not work one way, I will try another."

On a bright and blue-skied autumn morning, 21 exuberant fourth-graders came bursting into their classroom at Butler School in Springfield, IL. Their teacher, Miss Becky Murphy, was waiting for them. She enthusiastically braced herself for the outpouring of notes from home, fund-raiser forms, and proud presentations of home computer projects.

Just one year ago, Becky Murphy did not have the energy to get out of her hospital bed on the oncology unit of Springfield's Memorial Medical Center. Faced with a new diagnosis of acute leukemia, the popular grade school teacher suddenly found herself in the role of a student learning very difficult lessons.

Leukemia was a whole new world for Becky. Her life was filled with strange new medical terms and concerns. Instead of teaching her class writing and math skills, she had to learn about a disease process, daily blood counts, chemotherapy agents, antibiotics, and antifungals. Her treatment involved two months of hospitalization to put her leukemia in remission and two more months of intense outpatient intravenous antifungal therapy. Unfortunately, the treatments also seemed to put her mind in the same state. "I lost my memory. I even lost my ability to read," she said. "Teaching was the only thing I knew how to do."

Becky knew she had to get herself back in the classroom. She used her teaching skills to enhance her memory and reading ability. She took the advice that she had given to her students: Read as much as you can and practice your lessons. She read the same pages of her favorite books, including the Bible, every day until her memory started to come back.

When a student's parents came in at conference time and told her about their child's stubbornness, Becky could relate. She would say, "If they are stubborn, I am even more stubborn. I am here, aren't I? Stubborn is good. I have never given up on anything. I do not know how. I will not give up on my kids and I will not give up on myself. If something does not work one way, I will try another."

Becky continued, "I fought hard not to die, which is funny because there was a period before my cancer when I felt ready to die. I thought life was too hard; the world was too hard."

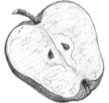

Looking back, Becky views her old complaints of asthma, allergies, and arthritis as trivial. "Priorities change with cancer," she explained. She was shocked at the support she found in her doctors, nurses, friends, fellow teachers, and former students.

"I came to realize that I was not ready to die," she said. "Now I realize that it is wonderful to live."

Sue Dinges, RN
Staff nurse on an oncology unit
Illinois

So, I have been put back in the position of beginner, looking at things with a beginner's eyes. It has lightened my load tremendously. It has given me an appreciation for new things that come my way.

Deborah Adam
Breast cancer survivor
Ohio

Cancer "unhinged" my ordinary perception of life and allowed me to become a doorway into myself. I have found many things there . . . inside. I have learned to live in the present—that's all any of us ever has. All that humanity has experienced, and all that will be, is here now. . . . Revel in the moment!

Libbie Kerr
Three-year breast cancer survivor
Ohio

Prayer From Camp Bluebird

"My mom is my hero." —John William Watson
(Rosemary Talbott's son)

Tennessee Camp Bluebird, sponsored by Saint Thomas Hospital and Telephone Pioneers of America, is a unique experience for adults with cancer. The three-day, two-night camp is held each spring and fall. Its purpose is to provide a time for listening, learning, caring, and sharing. It also is an opportunity to explore lessons of adjustments in living with cancer and how to give, receive, and ask for family support. The following is a prayer from this camp experience.

Dear Lord,
Thank You for another day,
Within this life of mine.
Let me live it well,
Whatever I may find.
Bestow from Thy abundance,
Whatever I may lack,
To use the hours wisely,
For I cannot have them back.

Lord, thank You for another day,
In which to make amends.
For the little slights or petty words,
Inflicted on my friends,
For sometimes losing patience,
With problems that I find.

Lord, thank You for another chance.
To show Your love is kind.
For yesterday is over,
And tomorrow's far away,
And I remained committed,
To do the good I do today.

Rosemary Talbott, LPN
Mother of four and soon-to-be grandmother of five, hospital chaplain,
oncology licensed practical nurse, and cancer survivor
Tennessee

From Black and White to Full Color

I reflect on the fact that I almost died to show me how much I really wanted to live!

Before my diagnosis of leukemia, I struggled with depression. At times I felt it would be better to die than to live with the depression, mistrust, and anger. I felt bitterness toward everything. Most of the time I was in denial. Only my family and close friends knew of my despair.

Something happened to me when I was told, "You have leukemia." Everyone I personally knew who had leukemia had died. Suddenly, I wanted to live! The very doctor in whom I had confided about my depression and despair said, "This reminds me of the story *It's a Wonderful Life*." I finally realized that there are so many great things about life. I fought very hard to live. My usual negative outlook turned to positive energy. I focused on getting well.

I realized how many people cared about me when I received hundreds of cards and baskets of flowers and well wishes. My relationships with others—my husband, family, and friends—have greatly improved in quality. Perhaps the most significant change is my renewed trust in the Lord. I always felt I had to be in control. Quite honestly, I had a difficult time trusting and turning my life over to Him. I learned the positive effects of the power of prayer firsthand, and placing my trust, without reservation, in the Lord made a difference for me. I have grown spiritually and have a stronger faith now. I reflect on the fact that I almost died to show me how much I really wanted to live!

Although we have had some personal tragedies since then, I can effectively cope and put them in their proper perspective. It has been almost five years since my diagnosis and bone marrow transplant. My life has truly changed from black and white to full color.

Rosemary Bloom
Bone marrow transplant survivor
Ohio

Bonding Through Baldness

The love and hope inside are what make us special people.

What is it about hair that makes a person special? Some of us spend hours to make our locks beautiful. A day can be great or just simply awful depending entirely upon our hair!

What do you think it feels like to know your hair is all going to fall out? When I pictured that long, thick, curly hair coming out in the shower, I could imagine multiple calls to the plumber for clogged drains. So, I went to the beauty shop and had them cut my hair very short. I was ready—or so I thought. Nothing could ever prepare me for the real thing. In the morning, my pillow and bed were covered with hair. When I got out of the shower, my body was covered with hair. There was no end to it! It was falling out everywhere!

Thank heaven for my wonderful husband. When I told him I wanted to shave my head to get rid of what was left, he volunteered to help me. Using clippers and several disposable shavers, I was now totally bald. My husband said that if I was bald, he was going to be bald, too. He shaved his head. Later, I received a phone call from my son's fiancee in Virginia. She was in tears and hardly able to speak. "You will never guess what he has done," she uttered. "He shaved his head! We were supposed to have our engagement pictures taken! Will he have hair by the time of the wedding?" My oldest son, like his father, had shaved his head.

Wearing a wig or hat during the summer in Florida is an experience. I never knew my head could sweat so much. I decided that going bald—no wig or hat—was usually the more desirable option, even if people stared. One day, however, while I was at a local store trying on dresses, I wore a hat. I carefully put it on in front of the three-fold mirror each time I left the changing room. The last dress I put on seemed to fit particularly well, and looks and stares from other patrons seemed to confirm that this was the best choice. Suddenly, it dawned on me that the looks and stares were at my bald head—I had forgotten to wear my hat.

My husband, my son, and I all now have hair. It's not important anymore. The love and hope inside are what make us special people.

Karen Sondregger
Nurse and breast cancer survivor
Florida

Turning Up the Volume

Cells regenerate, hair grows back,
and the spirit endures.

When I was diagnosed with breast cancer in October of 1994, I did not imagine there could ever be a silver lining to such a devastating experience. All I knew was that cancer represented loss and heartache. This diagnosis thrust me into a new reality where fear ruled and any semblance of control that I thought I had over my life seemed to be gone for good.

Cancer was cruel. Just 21 months earlier, my older sister had died of breast cancer. Suddenly, at age 41, I found myself facing the same nightmare. Cancer took part of my body and shook my confidence. I had been in a custody battle for my five-year-old son in a divorce case just prior to my diagnosis. I fought for my son and I won. Now I had to fight for my life.

I was petrified when told that I would require both chemotherapy and radiation. I was especially terrified at the prospect of losing my hair. I bought a wig to wear until it grew back and attended a *Look Good . . . Feel Better* program. I had some very low days following my treatments, but through the worst of it, I slowly began to glimpse the other side of cancer . . . not just one but many silver linings.

Cancer tested both my physical and my spiritual strength. I turned to God in prayer, and I was not disappointed. Cancer forced me to stop everything I was doing and redirect my priorities. Whereas I initially viewed this as an unfair interruption of my life, I finally realized that it was only God's way of "turning up the volume"—of forcing me to listen to His message to make positive changes and to let go of the painful divorce. I learned to set aside career pressures and focus on what is really important. I had to heal myself. Cancer provided the opportunity. This realization—cancer as opportunity—was my first ray of silver lining.

I found my second silver lining in all the people who sustained me then and continue to support me now. When I think of the resources and love expended to keep me alive and well, I am amazed and humbled by the value others have placed on my life. Cancer makes it impossible to take for granted an act of love, a word of kindness, or a gesture of support. Out of sheer need, you draw on this reservoir to keep going. I feel blessed by many loved ones: my family, doctors, nurses, pastor, attorney, and friends. All offered words of comfort, encouragement, and prayer. Their love created a silver lining of special radiance.

Random silver linings also came along to surprise me. When I needed protection from the sun, I went shopping for a straw hat and a stranger commented on how good I looked in hats. The compliment was so unexpected, I could not help but smile. My greatest silver lining, however, is my little boy. He is too young to really understand what I have been experiencing, but from the beginning he has been my motivation to keep going. My lengthy convalescence kept me at home and afforded us precious time together.

I don't wish to be misunderstood. Even though I am happy to have learned some valuable lessons, had the choice been mine, I would not have chosen cancer as my teacher. I would not want to trivialize the cancer experience in any way or to leave the impression that I blithely ignore its aftermath, or even that I have conquered the fear. I still believe that cancer is cruel and senseless. It changes you forever, but if you are open, you can take something back. Cells regenerate, hair grows back, and the spirit endures. Even my sister is with me still in cherished memories and the bond of love we shared. Hope can replace fear. Therein lies the secret to the silver linings. I am no longer merely a victim or a patient. I am a survivor!

Antoinette Castiglie-Falciano
Mother, friend, family member, and breast cancer survivor
New York

My son was nine months old when melanoma got me. Now he's three-and-one-half years old. Every night when I go to bed, I thank God I'm his mother. Every morning when I awake, I look at my son and realize how much of life I could have missed for a tan.

Janette Lamerson
Mother, nurse, and malignant melanoma survivor
Ohio

Celebrate the Memories

Life is a fiesta. We need to dance to our individual song that comes from the deepest part of our beings.

Cancer begins silently. There is no warning in day-to-day existence. Suddenly it blossoms from some routine test or unusual symptom, and then your world turns inside out. The disease influences everything you do—no matter what treatment course you take. Who are you? Everything looks different in your world: your friends, your family, your job, sunshine and rain, who you were before, who you are now, and, most importantly, who you will be in the future.

Yes, each day has changed. Only what is tied to the heart becomes important. As a cancer survivor, I can say this in many different ways. As an oncology nurse and a poet, I have said it even before my own cancer. Now I ask, "Where is the silver lining?" Is it the lining of a bright, sun-shining day? Is it cool silver metal? Does it line the darkness of moon-held dreams? For me, it became all of this as I relearned everything that I had previously told my patients in daily encounters. My words took on new meaning as my patients noticed my wig and my new-found understanding. Coworkers also shared my expertise and first-hand experiences with cancer to their patients. I became an expert in an area where I thought I was already proficient. This expertise began to go outward to patients—similar to the ripples in a pond when a stone is thrown in. Patients with cancer knew I understood all aspects of their disease. In the process, my coworkers also benefitted as they watched me continue to work through treatment. We all became stronger for it.

CELEBRATE THE MEMORIES
Celebrate the times of laughter,
the holding of hands,
the sharing of the hug between friends,
the child's soft kiss on your cheek.
Remember good times
and let them brighten each day.

Life is a fiesta. We need to dance to our individual song that comes from the deepest part of our beings. When the sad times come, wear the dark colors to accent the brighter moments and then let them go. If we hold on to them, they will tarnish the very depths of our soul. This is the lesson I learned—even though I thought I knew it before. Suddenly it became vital to my being.

LIFE IS A FIESTA
Wear sunlight colors in your heart.
Imagine the Southern wind combing your hair
and let your eyes dance with a summer light.
In the celebration of each day
dress laughter with morning waking.
Let night fold moonlight with stars
that reflect all prisms of color in your dreams.

Christine Umscheid, RN
Breast cancer survivor and oncology nurse
Michigan

The gifts of cancer nursing: to see the human spirit, emotions, courage, bravery, suffering, and healing—up close and personal. These gifts are what make it worthwhile.

Jennifer Gougas, RN, BSN, OCN®
Oncology nurse
California

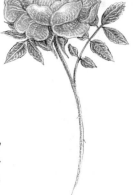

In the nine years that have passed since I underwent treatment for testicular cancer, four children have become prominent in my life. Through them I have recaptured my youth. I thank the Lord for the opportunity to "teach them to sing in perfect harmony."

David Stanley
Testicular cancer survivor
California

Desires of the Heart

*My goal was to grow old with my husband and to watch my teenage
daughters grow to adulthood with careers and families of their own.
These were the desires of my heart.*

I appreciate every day and every moment to the fullest because God
loves me enough to keep me here on earth to fulfill His purpose for me.
At 37, I was too young to have breast cancer! The reality was that I did
have cancer, and survival became the greatest challenge of my life.
Surgery, radiation, and chemotherapy did not daunt my will to survive.
This cancer journey demanded a thorough examination of my soul. My
husband, daughters, family, friends, and coworkers were my network of
care and support. My oncologist encouraged me to actively participate
in the decisions of my care and treatment. I also received spiritual
support from my church and many prayer lists from across the nation.

My goal was to grow old with my husband and to watch my teenage
daughters grow to adulthood with careers and families of their own.
These were the reasons to live each day and strive for tomorrow.

My hair has grown back, including the gray, and I have found a wonderful hairdresser, Judy. I have returned to work and continue working on my PhD. I try to live each day to the fullest. I strive to
always embrace life to the fullest, take the good with the bad, and
achieve the desires of the heart.

Kathy White
Intensive care nurse and metastatic breast cancer survivor
Georgia

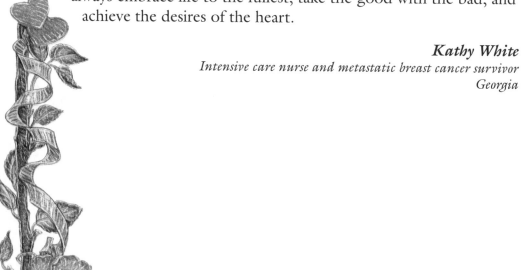

A Blessing in Disguise

Cancer brought me to my senses and jolted me into a renewed realization of life's fragility and goodness. I was reminded that my most cherished blessings continue to be family, friends, faith, and laughter.

Breast cancer has been a blessing in my life. No, I am not a victim of some type of severe chemotherapy overdose! I certainly would have opted out of the cancer sweepstakes if I had been given a choice. However, within a few months of my 40th birthday, cancer became a reality in my life. I suddenly found myself facing the experience, complete with a mastectomy and six months of chemotherapy. I survived with much support from family, friends, and members of my religious community, as well as the precious gifts of humor and faith.

Humor took many forms. For instance, my friends made tasteless jokes about double-breasted suits and suggested that I view my hair loss as "gaining face." Humor also helped me endure even the worst side effects. One book suggested viewing nausea as a positive sign that chemotherapy was working. The idea stuck with me. I still laugh as I recall clinging to the toilet bowl muttering, "Gosh, it is working!"*

The faith that my mother had instilled in me also played a key role in my recovery. Though often frightened, I never doubted that I would survive. I believed that God would give me the strength to endure . . . and God did. It was as simple and mysterious as that.

My encounter with cancer undoubtedly has been the most profound experience of my life. Cancer brought me to my senses and jolted me into a renewed realization of life's fragility and goodness. I was reminded that my most cherished blessings continue to be family, friends, faith, and laughter. Indeed, cancer has been a blessing in my life.

Susan Bremer, OSU
Breast cancer survivor
Ohio

* *Editors' note:* The amount of nausea one experiences has no relevance to the effectiveness of the treatment.

Thinking of You in Kalamazoo

Cancer takes ordinary people and teaches them to be extraordinary.

My days are no longer ordinary. They are bright and full of new and exciting things. It is sad to realize that the life I took for granted had to be threatened before I realized just how precious each day is.

Two years ago, I heard the doctor say *the word*: "Val, you have *cancer*." Immediately, death entered my mind. But with faith, and a significant attitude readjustment, I turned something completely devastating into a positive experience and a lesson in life. I put my Dutch-Irish heritage into gear and faced eight chemotherapy and 33 radiation treatments. I had very few days when I did not smile.

So, with my new bald head, I decided to dress in a costume for Halloween. When I walked into the West Michigan Cancer Center that day, I noticed a few stunned faces. The women in the lab asked, "Val, what are you doing?"

"Trick or treating for my chemotherapy, and you may trick or treat out of my basket," I replied while offering my goodies.

I visited the other patients who were at the center for their chemotherapy and let them take a Halloween treat out of my basket. In actuality, I not only brought smiles to others that day but also made myself feel good!

Like many other survivors, patients with cancer share a special bond. We have "been there and done that." We know what it is like. I continue to dress up in my silly getups and visit the West Michigan Cancer Center on holidays. A year ago, I met a gentleman who asked me for a gun so he would not have to suffer any more. However, before I left that day, his hand was in mine. Two days later, he called to thank me. Whether he knows it or not, he gave me so much more than I gave him that day.

My message to the reader with cancer is that there is a light at the end of the tunnel. You must have faith, hope, and lots of humor! When I go to bed at night, I thank God for the life

He has given back to me. I pray for all of you who share this disease with me. My life is full and I am grateful for those people who support me. To my children, Amy and Michael, my special friend, Walt, and the staff at West Michigan Cancer Center, know that I love you with all my heart! To all of you who read this, remember that, no matter how far away you are, you have a friend in Kalamazoo with a survival hug just for you! God Bless!

Valarie J. Jansen
Survivor and lover of life
Michigan

Sheheheyanu
Thank you to illness, to cancer
Teacher of lessons otherwise unlearned
The gift of dark days
Of fear and waiting and the unknown
Awakening on the other side
To the miracle of appreciation
Of just being alive each new day
How short and fragile life is
How precious each breath

Out of pain arises incredible joy
Wonder and awe at the miracle of the
Everyday ordinariness of life
I took so for granted before

Becoming a Bat Mitzvah
Is my way to say
Thank you, God
Sheheheyanu

Betsy Firger
Attorney, wife, and mother of three teenagers and
four-year survivor of non-Hodgkin's lymphoma
Connecticut

Wealth and Wisdom

The struggle of allowing others to help me and simply saying "thank you" was very difficult.

He could not be talking about me! I felt like I was having an out-of-body experience, soaring above the doctor and me. I listened to him tell me that I had a growth blocking my colon. Deep inside, I knew it was cancer. As a nurse, I could ignore the signs no longer. The mind is a powerful thing. It allows you to believe what you wish when the truth is too unbearable.

My symptoms had persisted for several months before I finally visited my gynecologist for a regular checkup. He asked me questions that I could not avoid answering. The result was a visit to a gastrointestinal specialist for what I hoped would be the diagnosis of internal hemorrhoids. I knew better, but I had hope. That was the day my journey with cancer began. This was a strange journey—terrifying at times, yet also rewarding in many ways. Who in their right mind could call the cancer experience rewarding? Allow me to explain.

My husband, Jim, and his family always have been extremely healthy. Even with his lack of medical knowledge, Jim knew as he looked at my face that something was terribly wrong. From the very beginning of this unplanned journey, Jim was my strength and best cheerleader. He studied the information on colon cancer that I had provided for him. Armed with information from the literature, he became my chief dietitian and master chef during my chemotherapy and radiation treatments. He continues to let me know, in so many ways, that a wife with a colostomy is still a treasure to him. He has repeated so many times that he is grateful that I am alive.

When my boss heard the news, she was right by my side with words of encouragement and assurance. She made it possible for me to work from home during my surgical recovery period. She always shared with me her confidence that I would beat this cancer and soon be back on the job. I never felt that my job was in jeopardy or that she would treat me any differently than before the diagnosis.

My coworkers also were supportive. Although I was able to work most of the time during my therapy, they assured me that they would pick up the work that I was unable to complete. They did just as they promised. I truly was part of a team that cared for one another, and they felt my recovery was important. Just knowing how hard my coworkers were working for me helped me return to work sooner.

I was concerned about telling my mother, who is in her 80s, about the long road that lay ahead of me. She was recovering from her own major surgery and coping with my father's deteriorating health condition. I discovered that my mother is a woman of substance. She was, and continues to be, a great source of strength. She insisted on nursing me back to health after my surgery.

Another amazing grace that I experienced was the realization that so many people loved me and wanted me to live. I expected my family to love me, but not the hundreds of other people who also professed their love. The amount of cards and flowers that came was astounding. The prayers that were said for me in churches of all religions were powerful. As never before, I believe that the power of prayer is the most significant force that affected my outcome.

I have always been an independent person. I was accustomed to doing for others and being the Supermom and the hardest-working employee. I seldom allowed others to assist me. The struggle of allowing others to help me and simply saying "thank you" was very difficult. I remember feeling so frustrated when my husband and close friends organized a house-decorating party so Christmas would be preserved in the style to which I was accustomed. They did not do things as I would have done; however, as I watched them decorating, I realized how blessed I was to have them, and I noticed their joy at being able to do something tangible for me. I now allow people to love me by their actions. In return, I have learned to hug them and tell them how much I appreciate them.

Perhaps now you can understand that, even in the darkest of times, rewarding experiences can be found. My approach to life is different since I began this journey with cancer. Now I greet each day with the pleasure of being alive. I thank God for how He has shaped my life. I have a great job, extraordinary coworkers, supportive friends, a loving family, and the most wonderful husband in the world. Yes, I am a cancer survivor . . . and I am a rich woman!

Ivette Carver
Nurse and cancer survivor
Florida

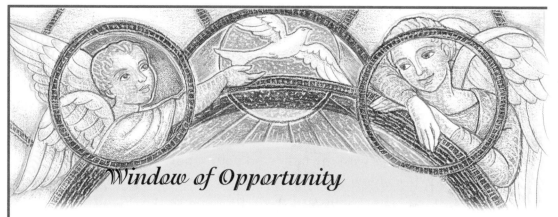

Window of Opportunity

My cancer was a gift. A time to see my life anew. A time to get off the carousel of the routine and appreciate the awesomeness and newness of every day, every moment—each so different from the next.

"Behind every door that closes, a window opens." This, or something quite like it, is what a fond, Irish poet friend of mine said to me upon hearing I had cancer. When he did, I thought it was mostly a crock of potato-field Irish blarney. But over the next six months of my chemo-therapy and recovery, his words came back to me many a time.

I was diagnosed with Hodgkin's disease on April 7, 1989. I remember the date. It was my sister's birthday. I had been feeling sick for months, but never did I imagine that it might be cancer. Sometimes I would think I was imagining the pain—sharp, floating stabs in my sides, then in my back, then in my abdomen, followed by nothing—no pain. All the tests were negative for gall bladder disease, kidney stones, and irritable bowel. I figured it was nothing more than stress or hypochondria.

Six frustrating months later, I finally was referred to the right doctor, a smart and gentle oncologist. Recognizing all the symptoms I reported—night sweats, itchy skin, internal pain—he suggested I go for a biopsy. He didn't push me, he didn't panic—he simply suggested. I hardly knew what a biopsy was, but I went, more to eliminate the possibility of anything else. The next day, Saturday, April 7, he called me to tell me that he was sorry that the results were positive. I had a cancer of the lymphatic system called Hodgkin's disease.

I couldn't believe it. I was in complete shock! It couldn't be. Little ol' me with the big bad *C*? Impossible! I freaked. I couldn't tell anyone, not even my parents or my sister, Alison. When I called to wish her a happy birthday, I didn't mention anything about it. A week or so later, I finally had a close friend with another life-threatening illness call my folks and tell them for me. When I spoke to them a few days later, I could hear the fear in their voices. I immediately started to take care of them, urging them not to worry. I instantly knew that I did not want them to come to Los Angeles to "take care of me." I needed this time to take care of myself.

With the diagnosis of cancer, I felt the door close on the first 42 years of my life. Slowly, however, a window began to open. What started with fear, panic, and denial ended up with love, forgiveness, and self-acceptance. You see, I discovered I had a choice—a choice between closing up and fearing life or opening up and living fully. I chose the latter. I chose to live in the moment, day by day—to appreciate what I had in my life instead of what I didn't have. I learned to give and accept love more freely. I put down my sword and shield, my anger and ambition. I picked up gratitude and surrender, appreciation and spontaneity. Maybe I didn't have a choice. Perhaps because of the severity of the illness and the harshness of the treatment, living one day at a time was all I could do. Life was an emotional roller coaster—full of ups and downs, pains, and releases. I ate like a pig, and I starved. I cried and laughed, raged and gave thanks—every day. My life was never so full.

My cancer was a gift. A time to see life anew. A time to get off the carousel of the routine and appreciate the awesomeness and newness of every day, every moment—each so different from the next. Unbelievably, even in retrospect, I can honestly say that the time of my illness was the happiest time in my life. Yes, the treatment was an ordeal. Yes, at one time I was so afraid of dying that I couldn't fall asleep. But ultimately, my cancer was a window of opportunity, a chance to reconsider and reappreciate the wonder of life. They say that only those faced with the finality of death can appreciate the transitory and fragile nature of life.

Someone reading this may still be on the other side, looking at the closed door of a cancer diagnosis, perhaps facing a prognosis less promising than mine with Hodgkin's. I encourage you to go deeper inside yourself and to look for that open window. I know it's there. Look for it everyday. I'm grateful to have made it through remission and cure. I'm a survivor. Yet, I remember that my greatest joy and satisfaction came when I was smiling through that window of opportunity.

Eric Trules
Poet, filmmaker, and Hodgkin's disease survivor
California

Ordinary Days Equal an Extraordinary Life

*Cancer brought me closer to my family. It forced me to
rethink my value system.*

Looking back on the five years since I was diagnosed and treated
for colorectal cancer, I have no doubts that the experience changed
my life. Cancer brought me closer to my family. It forced me to
rethink my value system. It caused me to appreciate the pieces of life
that I previously had taken for granted.

The most immediate and obvious change that I experienced was
my relationship with my family. Cancer brought my family together
for physical and emotional aid. I was only 24 years old and living
alone with no family living nearby. My parents and brothers pulled
together and provided support by staying with me, preparing meals,
encouraging me to work part-time, and driving me to and from
treatments for six months. The most important gift they gave me,
however, was laughter and a reason to keep my chin up. They kept
me going.

At the time of my diagnosis, I had just graduated from college and
started a new job in Cleveland, Ohio. Most of my friends were making similar choices—high-paying jobs with large companies in urban
areas. The high salary was very important to us so we could buy
everything we needed: new cars, trendy clothes, entertainment, and
evenings out. I, too, was caught up in what I now call the "preten-
tious world." I look back on those days and find I have little toler-
ance for that life-style and image. I realized this one day while shopping with a friend. Prior to my illness, we had spent hours trying on
and buying nice clothing in expensive shops. It suddenly occurred to
me that putting a great deal of time and money into a wardrobe just
was not me anymore.

Instead, I take time to notice and appreciate events that occur in
small moments each normal day. So what if my car wouldn't start or
the washing machine leaked. It's still a good day to me—because I
am alive and because I spent a few moments with a purring cat or
planted my sugar-snap peas. Realistically, I have a work schedule and
cannot meander through each day. I have realized the importance of
building time into each day for solitude, relaxation, and exercise. Of

course, I look forward to that perfect vacation coming up soon, but I also look forward to today, tonight, and tomorrow.

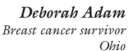

Linda Laney
Age 29; treated for colorectal cancer in 1992
Indiana

Each day is a miracle in itself, for me to observe and experience. The distractions of the world keep us from appreciating the joy that is now.

Deborah Adam
Breast cancer survivor
Ohio

Life is "normal" again, and each day is a gift to be cherished. Going through a bone marrow transplant has been my hardest trial. However, it also has proved to be my greatest strength. The need to write about my experiences has been the greatest source of healing. The learning and growth must never be forgotten.

Analisa O'Rullian
Eight-year survivor of
bone marrow transplant for leukemia
California

 Focus on the moment—for moments are what make up our lives. Live in the moment, be present in the present, be grateful to be alive.

Dawn Stobbe
Ovarian cancer survivor
Nebraska

There Is Life After Breast Cancer

Breast cancer is just a diagnosis. It does not limit me or define me as a person.

On January 2, 1994, just two weeks past my 31st birthday, I was diagnosed with breast cancer. It was a shock to me because I always thought of breast cancer as a grandmother's disease—certainly not something I had to worry about. How wrong I was. I learned firsthand that breast cancer doesn't choose you by your age, race, or social status. I never thought of myself as a strong person before. Yet, when I heard my diagnosis, I was determined not to die while I had two small children to raise and future grandchildren to see. I was angry that this disease invaded my body without my consent. I was determined that I would do all I could to keep it out of my body.

I had many tears and a great deal of anger to deal with. I'll never forget when my hair began to fall out. I quickly grabbed a can of hair spray in hopes that it would hold it in place. Imagine the money the hair spray company would be making today if it had held up against hair loss from chemotherapy! When my hair loss progressed, my son Eric (age six) thought it was pretty cool that his mom looked better bald than the old neighbor across the street. Humor has always played a leading role in my fight against breast cancer.

Now I consider my breast cancer a mixed blessing. I feel that only those of us who are in this "sisterhood" truly understand what I mean by this. Although I believe that no one really wants to face their own mortality, if we are wise we will know we have been given a special gift. It has been three years now since my diagnosis, and in that time, I feel that I have grown into a better person. I try to help others by talking with them and by participating in community projects. I will continue to volunteer until people no longer say, "But, you are too young to have breast cancer." You see, it still bothers me that so many people believe that this is a disease for older women. Some women younger than I am have this disease.

I want others to look at me without pity. I want others to know that breast cancer is just a diagnosis. It does not define or limit me as a person. There *is* life after breast cancer, and it is a good life! Each day is special and a gift. I wake up each morning knowing that I am ready to face and handle anything.

Tish Johnson
Wife, mother of two small boys, and breast cancer survivor
Nebraska

I have been a survivor for almost two years. After a mastectomy and six months of chemotherapy, the roller coaster began to slow down. I started to realize that work would survive without me. If the house did not get cleaned, the health department would not come and shut it down. I still have my moments. I really haven't accepted the way I look. But each day that I am able to wake up and smell the coffee is one more day I have to treasure the love and the friendships in my life.

Renee Behrens
Breast cancer survivor
Illinois

As a seven-year breast cancer survivor, I can truly say there have been more positives than negatives. As I continue my journey of cancer survivorship, I will continue to have a greater appreciation of life until I reach my final destination.

Deanna A. Beyer, MS, RN
Seven-year breast cancer survivor
Michigan

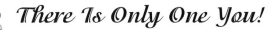

There Is Only One You!

If I worry about tomorrow, then I have lost today. Illness is a great teacher. I have learned to be kinder to myself.

I was diagnosed with breast cancer at age 34. As a result, both of my breasts were removed and reconstructed with silicone implants. I experienced metastasis to multiple spots on the spine and other bones. This past spring, I learned that the cancer had spread to my ovaries, fallopian tubes, and omentum. Over the years, I have had several rounds of chemotherapy, including high-dose chemotherapy with an autologous bone marrow transplant, several surgeries, and radiation.

Since the very beginning of this journey, I became my own patient advocate. I read as much as I could and asked many questions, especially when I did not understand what was happening. I changed doctors when I felt it was necessary. I encouraged other patients to ask questions or to get more information. The physician's job is to tell you what is happening, what to expect from the treatment, and what the treatment hopefully will achieve.

If you have any doubts about your doctor's recommendations, get another opinion. A second opinion either will confirm your doubts or give you more confidence. Please remember that your doctors may be brilliant and wonderful, but they also are treating hundreds of other patients. Seek information on appropriate new treatments and make suggestions to your doctor. By taking an active role in your treatment decisions, you will be helping yourself and your physician. Remember, there is *only one you* and that is the person you should be concerned with.

Ironically, cancer has been somewhat of a blessing in my life. I have learned to appreciate life so much more. Each day is special, and I try to live in the moment. What happened in the past does not matter to me now. If I worry about tomorrow, then I have lost today. I have learned to be kinder to myself. I make time to do things that I enjoy. I have found massages to be helpful. They improve circulation, help eliminate toxins in the body, and relax tense muscles. Acupuncture has been beneficial as a means of pain control. Visualization and meditation have been helpful in my fight for recovery as well. I also have explored psychic and Reiki healers, but only as an addition to traditional medicine.

Do whatever it takes—physically, emotionally, and spiritually—to help yourself heal. We may never know why we were afflicted with cancer, but what's important is how we deal with it. Illness can be a great teacher.

Sandra P. DeSalvo
Twelve-year breast cancer survivor
Ohio

My life has permanently changed. The catalyst? Cancer. No longer do I take for granted a beautiful, star-filled night, a rose's delicacy, the quiet rapport that exists between my loved ones and me, nor the joy of being alive and healthy one more day.

Dolores Cornejo, LCSW
Breast cancer survivor and
pediatric oncology social worker
California

Each day dawns with hope and wonder in God, in others, and in life! I am not the same person I was a year ago. More important than being free from cancer, I have freed myself to become the beautiful, human creation God desires me to be— rather than the uptight, "perfect" person I had been.

Bobbie Donahue
Cancer survivor
Nebraska

Carolyn's Story

I have learned to love life and never take it for granted.

My cancer was like being reborn and starting a new and different life. My family and I will soon be celebrating my third year being cancer-free. It is a big day for all of us. I will have three candles on my cake. I will be filled with happiness and will shed tears. The tears are not sad ones. Instead, they are tears of joy.

I am so thankful to God for giving me life, and I plan to live it to the fullest. I see beauty in all the seasons—yes, even in the cold, blowing snows of a Nebraska winter. I have learned to love life and never take it for granted. For me, all the feelings I have experienced came together and are expressed in the following poem I wrote.

> If I were a bird, I could sing so pretty
> If I were the sun, I could shine so bright
> If I were a flower, I could stand so grateful
>
> I am not a bird, the sun, or a flower
> But I am a Cancer Survivor
> And thank God that
> I can hear the birds
> I can feel the sun
> I can see the flowers

Carolyn Sudyka
Three-year breast cancer survivor
Nebraska

For you, I wish many things—the love of family and friends, the gift of laughter, strength, courage, and wisdom. Most of all, I wish you peace—with yourself and your world.

Jean Loving, RN
Hospice/oncology volunteer and four-year
breast cancer survivor
North Carolina

Quest for the Silver Linings

*Cancer's silver lining is that it fuels our hunt for
other silver linings more intensely than ever.*

Some of my serendipitous silver linings surface when I least expect them. I saw a vixen and her three kits alongside the Alcan Highway en route to Alaska. I learned to snorkel so I could discover a polka-dotted tropical fish in the Virgin Islands National Park. While hiking in Alaska, I saw a moose and her wobbly-legged calf just four feet from me on the other side of a bush as they grazed. I was astounded by how huge they are when you are so close to them. It was a thrilling silver lining to see a quiet fawn mid-meadow just 20 feet from my trail. Through my binoculars, it looked like it was only a few feet away from me!

These silver linings *seem* serendipitous; yet, I take a good share of credit for creating them. Fortunately, my mother taught me early the quest for silver linings. I view it as both a skill and a mental attitude. It is a great arrow to have in your quiver when you take aim at cancer!

Cancer's wake-up call has accelerated my explorations and reconnected me with a wealth of warm, but widely scattered, family and friends. It has deepened my spirituality and helped me to finally do the unthinkable: write a book. I want to share my scheme for living zestfully and intentionally. I do have some novel ideas, such as why wait for the conception of my as-yet-unborn grandchildren, when that will be too late for me? I'm knitting some crib blankets and sweaters for them now!

Silver linings and seeming serendipity are a lot like good luck: They are very much our own doing and thinking. Cancer's silver lining is that it fuels our hunt for other silver linings more intensely than ever.

Laura A. Cross
Six-and-one-half-year breast cancer survivor
Texas, Michigan, New York, and North Carolina

*Today is someday. I can't have dreams that
I can put off. I must do things now.*

Denise Miner-Williams, RN, MSN
Registered nurse
Texas

On Your Mark, Get Set, Go!

Today I do not run. I walk and enjoy the view of life!

Actually, I do not even remember anyone blowing the whistle, but I was off and running as fast as I could. I thought I could have it all—a career, a loving husband, two adorable children, a nice house, great vacations, and community involvement. I was trying to live my entire life before the age of 40. After all, my mother had died of breast cancer when she was 39. In my early 30s, I heard a cancer surgeon speak at a meeting. The only words I remembered were, "If you have a strong family history, do not bury your head in the sand." So, I began my bi-yearly visits to the oncologist.

I quietly tiptoed through my 40th birthday—no parties, no fanfare. Then, during a routine breast examination, the oncologist noticed a swelling in my right breast. The mammogram appeared normal; however, while performing an aspiration, the doctor became suspicious. A subsequent lumpectomy confirmed my gut feeling. I had breast cancer. I chose to have a bilateral mastectomy followed by chemotherapy. My quality of life was more important to me than having two breasts!

After the chemotherapy treatments, my stomach became distended, but I assumed that it was only a side effect of the chemotherapy. Then I lost the feeling in my upper left thigh. I decided to visit my internist for a checkup. Upon seeing me, she promptly scheduled an x-ray. That evening, my gynecologist performed an ultrasound and confirmed that I had ovarian cancer.

Within five days, I underwent a complete hysterectomy and began a new cycle of chemotherapy.

Within 15 months, I was diagnosed with two different stage I cancers, had two major surgeries, and underwent 18 treatments of chemotherapy. I feel extremely fortunate to be alive! My priorities are now in proper perspective—family, diet and exercise, relaxation, spirituality, career, and community service. I now take time to practice Tai Chi, do polarity therapy, learn more about herbs, and attend a weekly religious class. Today I do not run. I walk and enjoy the view of life!

Wendy Avner
Breast and ovarian cancer survivor
Ohio

Learning to Love

Albert Schweitzer said it best when he wrote, "I don't know what your destiny will be, but one thing I do know: the only ones among you who will be really happy are those who have sought and found how to serve."

Prior to my bone marrow transplant for chronic myelogenous leukemia, I saw the world though a single eye. I looked only in the direction I chose and had no regard for those around me. I saw this as normal, healthy, and American. I was 28 years old, recently married, and living very comfortably. I thought I had it all. I've come to find out, however, I had so very much to learn.

Dealing with the difficulties of cancer shifts one's thoughts away from the material things in life to what is truly important. I now know that I am a part of those around me. What I give out, in the form of kind words, thoughts, and deeds, comes back to me, although that is not my reason for sharing. My responsibility as a human being is to help others, which inevitably helps all of us. I truly know now that unconditional love is the only true love. It is to be shared with everyone as often as possible.

Albert Schweitzer said it best when he wrote, "I don't know what your destiny will be, but one thing I do know: the only ones among you who will be really happy are those who have sought and found how to serve." This I learned through my struggles with this disease we call cancer. I will keep it with me for the rest of my life.

Kim Tolnar
Bone marrow transplant survivor
Ohio

Time is a precious gift.

Linda Battiato, RN, MSN, OCN®
Oncology nurse
Indiana

Anonymous Charity

As the bright red lifeline flows
To my pale, whitish arm by IV,
Giving me back my breath, my color, my energy—
Giving me back my life.

You gave your own blood;
Available only from your own body—
Totally irreplaceable.
Your gift of giving blood is
The ultimate mitzvah.

Anonymous charity—
Never knowing my face,
Never knowing my story,
Never knowing who will receive
This precious gift of life.

Your blood is sustaining me,
Keeping me alive,
Allowing me to reach this season.
My eyes fill with tears of awe and gratitude.
Thank you for saving my life.

How can I say thank you?
All I know you by is
Our shared blood type—
B Positive.
A good motto for life—
Be Positive!

Betsy Firger
Attorney, wife, and mother of three teenagers
and four-year survivor of non-Hodgkin's lymphoma
Connecticut

Eighty Years Young

While our heads are crowned with silver hair, our lives are full of gratitude—"lined" with silver for all these 21 bonus years of precious life and answered prayers.

A diagnosis of cancer strikes the heart and soul with fear and uncertainty. Cancer first touched our lives in 1975. My husband, Nick, responded to medication and radium treatments and did well. His bladder was replaced with what was then the newest internal conduit, which allowed him to be free of an external appliance. This was a miracle of convenience that allowed us to swim, fish, dance, travel, and enjoy activities with our children and grandchildren.

Our praises to our doctors and special nurses who encouraged us and taught me about Nick's care. We feel blessed to have this winning combination and our faith in God. Nick and I are 80 years young, and we have no doubts that while our heads are crowned with silver hair, our lives are full of gratitude —"lined" with silver for all these 21 bonus years of precious life and answered prayers.

Elena Helen Virca
Wife of cancer survivor
Ohio

My husband and I experienced great personal growth. We learned to let go and let God. We took a leap of faith [after I took chemotherapy and radiation] and decided to attempt another pregnancy. Miraculously, I was pregnant in three months! After the smoothest pregnancy with no morning sickness, I had a healthy baby girl, Jordyn Nicole Monroe. What a joy! We have received more blessings than we ever could have imagined.

Cynthia Monroe
Thriving four-year survivor
Ohio

Alive in HOPE

Alive to see children at play;
See another sunrise, sunset, one more day.
I awake, I pray,
Thank you, Lord, for blessing me with
another day.

Claire Forzano
Caretaker for husband who is a
prostate cancer survivor
New York

For now, it seems I can go on with my life
"as usual." The fact of the matter is, I do
not want to go on with my life "as usual." I
do not want to go back to the way things
were before my cancer. God has done too
many things in my heart, changed my
attitudes, changed my priorities, and given
me a new vision of each day to be lived fully
and joyfully. Cancer was a giant "wake-up
call" for me. How could I go back to how
things were before?

Janice L. Mahoney
Pastor's wife with breast cancer
Virginia

Each day when I wake, I touch my new,
beautiful, curly hair to make sure it is still
attached to my head. Then I smile. This
day belongs to me. That is enough.

Patricia L. Kinney
Breast cancer and bone marrow transplant
survivor, a.k.a. "Alive and well!"
Arizona

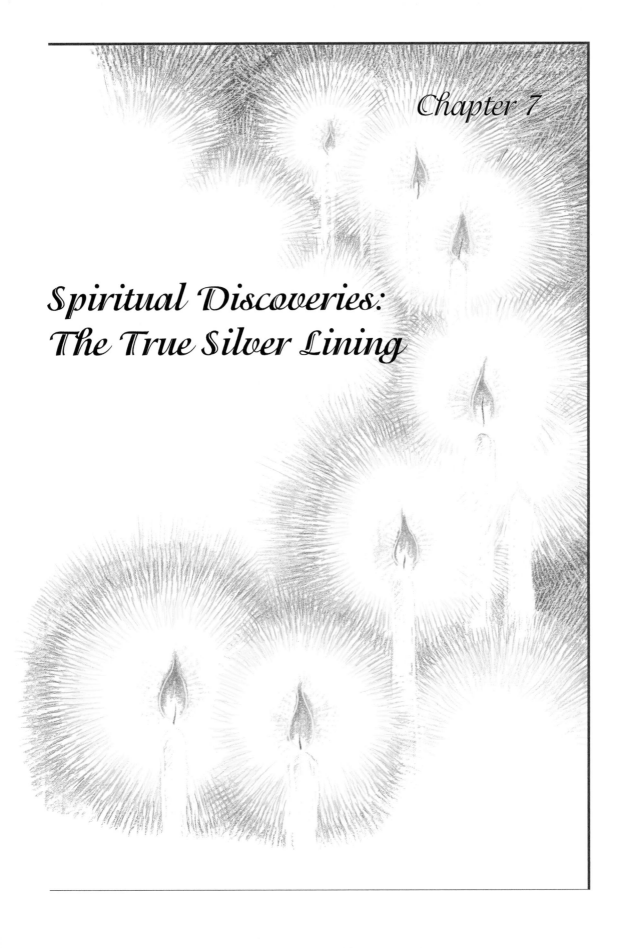

Chapter 7

Spiritual Discoveries: The True Silver Lining

Beyond the Tears

The important thing is to find ways to move beyond the initial negative reactions. Live life as fully as possible each day.

In early June 1995, I learned that I had a pancreatic tumor. This news took me totally by surprise. I had no symptoms of such an aggressive malignancy. I underwent radical surgery three days later. For the first time in my life, I had to directly face the prospect of a premature death. In one brief moment, my plans for the future were put on hold. Everything in my personal and ministerial life had to be reevaluated from a new perspective.

Naturally, I felt very vulnerable. However, my faith helped me to cope with the situation. I prayed as I never have prayed before that I would have the courage and grace to face whatever lay ahead. I then was blessed with an unparalleled peace of mind.

Nevertheless, I was not spared the anxiety and fear that such a diagnosis can cause. For example, during my convalescence after surgery, I often wept—something I seldom did before my cancer. I discovered that the cause of my tears was a fear that the cancer would return or my recovery would be incomplete. My ministry could be seriously affected as well. These reactions are part of the human condition and should be expected. So I made no effort to hide or deny them. The important thing is to find ways to move beyond the initial negative reactions. Live life as fully as possible each day.

Cardinal Joseph Bernardin
Illinois

Coming back from the brink of despair, I look to the future with the light of God on my shoulder. That is the peace that passes all understanding.

Margaret P. Barnhart
*Ten-year breast cancer survivor
and author of* Journey Unknown
Ohio

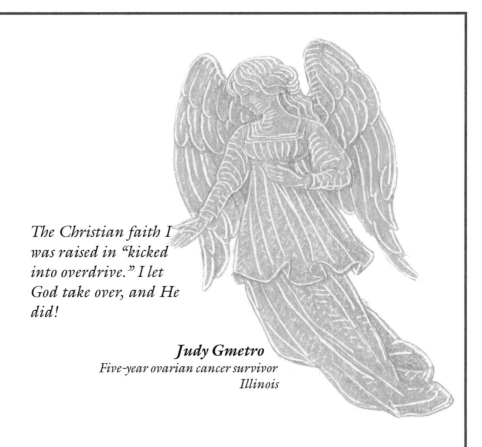

The Christian faith I was raised in "kicked into overdrive." I let God take over, and He did!

Judy Gmetro
Five-year ovarian cancer survivor
Illinois

I prayed to God,
"Father, I don't want to live like this.
I ask one of two things.
Would you heal me completely, or
would you take me home to Heaven?
I will accept what you want,
but I don't want to live like this."
After that, I felt an impression
on my heart as I prayed.
The impression was that
God would heal me.
I can't say I heard a voice—
but I felt an inner conviction.

Rev. Kenneth Schultz
Cancer survivor
Ohio

Feed Your Spirit

Cancer is a life-changing and attitude-changing wake-up call.

My father died of cancer two years ago, and my own cancer currently is in remission. I have experienced many precious, dear, and wonderful things since my diagnosis. However, they simply cannot be explained or fully conveyed to others unless they, too, have walked the valley of cancer and discovered the flowers in that valley.

My usual yearly mammogram in January 1996 revealed a suspicious area. I had a second mammogram. My doctor sent me to a surgeon for a biopsy, which confirmed three different types of cancer. I underwent a double mastectomy followed by chemotherapy because there was lymph node involvement. My blood count also fell dangerously low, so after I left the hospital I had daily injections of a medicine that forced the bone marrow to manufacture white blood cells. As with others who have had chemotherapy treatments, I experienced total hair loss, weakness, fatigue, susceptibility to infections, nausea, weight loss, headaches, bone pain, diarrhea, and vomiting. These are only the physical aspects of cancer; I have learned that there is so much more to life than the physical.

When the doctor said that frightening word, "cancer," I discovered my anchor. In this possible sentence of death, I had life. In this illness, I had spiritual health.

I realized that God is in control of all circumstances, even those that seem to be out of our control. I found comfort in Psalm 37:23–24: "The steps of a good man are ordered by the Lord: and he delighteth in His way. Though he falls, he will not be utterly cast down; for the Lord upholdeth him with His hand."

I learned how to have a joyful heart, no matter what was happening in my life. This advice I found in Proverbs 17:22: "A merry heart doeth good like a medicine; but a broken spirit drieth the bones."

I prayed often! I read and followed Philippians 4:6–7: "Be careful for nothing; but in everything be prayer and supplication with thanksgiving let your requests be made known unto God. And the peace of God, which passes all understanding, will keep your hearts and minds through Christ Jesus."

Cancer brings a depth of loving and a height of living that wasn't there before. Survivors do more than survive. We thrive.

Janice L. Mahoney
Pastor's wife and grandmother with breast cancer
Virginia

I rested in the Lord and reflected over my life with thanksgiving. Life has a deeper, new beginning.

Vernastine Kimble
Ordained minister, celebrating one year as a survivor of breast cancer
California

Sheila had a vital force all her own. She was transformed through her illness. I had never before seen the powers of belief affect biology. The potency of prayer and spiritual healing in treating cancer is awesome.

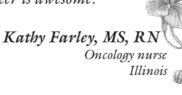

Kathy Farley, MS, RN
Oncology nurse
Illinois

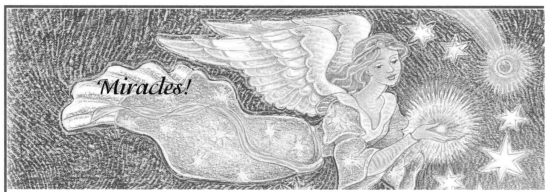

Miracles!

"Faith is the bird that feels the light and sings while the dawn is still dark." —Rabindranath Tagore

Miracles? I believe in them! The first patient I cared for after I graduated from nursing school taught me that they do happen. She was a 30-year-old woman who had just been diagnosed with acute myelogenous leukemia. She had a three-year-old and a six-month-old daughter. Over the next few months, I saw her through her chemotherapy, monitored her side effects, and taught her husband how to perform central catheter care. I held her hand through the loneliness of separation from her daughters and rejoiced with her about every good lab and bone marrow result. Many times we would be crying and laughing at the same time. Our laughter truly turned to tears when she developed intracranial bleeding resulting in stroke symptoms. The battle seemed lost. She got the news of the poor prognosis and the need for hospice care.

Months passed and the disease did not progress. In true heroic fashion, this wonderful lady set her sights on rehabilitation. She experienced some minor speech and cognitive deficits but was now able to care for her children. Time seemed the enemy now. I lost track of her when her husband's job caused them to move to several different states over the next few years. Occasionally a postcard would arrive at the oncologist's office letting us know of her whereabouts and how she was doing. We always posted them on our bulletin board as a form of inspiration to all of us.

Sixteen years later, I found myself working at the same hospice that had cared for her so many years before. And then came the day I will never forget. She walked into my office and said, "Hi! Remember me? My husband and I are working here as volunteers!" **Miracles do happen!**

Mary Murphy, RN, MS, OCN®
Oncology nurse
Ohio

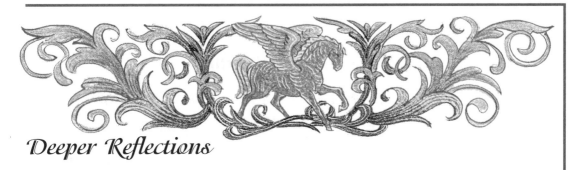

Deeper Reflections

I hope for kindness and peace wherever I am. I will do what I can to see that it is available to everyone.

"What good has come from having cancer?" Someone recently asked me this question at a support group meeting. My first response was, "I can't think of anything." However, deeper reflection has led me to the following conclusions.

1. Doctors are human. Their knowledge comes from years of study and experience. They do not always know what is best for me. The doctor and the patient must form a partnership and be completely honest with each other.

2. My spiritual life will weaken or strengthen, probably both. I may need to redefine answers I thought I already knew. I have faced death. I am satisfied that I have nothing to fear.

3. Others will not experience cancer the same way that I have experienced the disease. Others will not always say things that help me feel better. I can teach them what helps and what does not help if I so choose.

4. My health insurance company will not be my best friend, nor will we always agree. However, I would not want to face this illness without it.

5. I have learned to limit my commitments. I save my strength for things that are the most important in life.

6. Degrees and titles are nothing compared to the attitude and sensitivity of healthcare workers.

7. Cancer and its treatment have sent me far from where I was headed. I gained new respect for life and my relationships with others. I hope for kindness and peace wherever I am. I will do what I can to see that it is available to everyone.

Margaret P. Barnhart
Ten-year breast cancer survivor
and author of Journey Unknown
Ohio

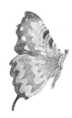

What Has Cancer Brought Me?

I couldn't die yet. I wanted to do something significant with my life—something I could be proud of.

In June 1990, at age 26, I was diagnosed with acute lymphocytic leukemia. After the shock wore off, I started thinking of all the things I still hadn't done in my life: things I thought I had plenty of time left for, things that I was always going to do tomorrow, or the next day. I couldn't die yet. I wanted to do something significant with my life— something I could be proud of. I prayed, asking God to please get me through this somehow. I promised that if He would give me one more year of life, I would make something of it. I wouldn't be just doing things I wanted to do but rather doing something for others for a change. I knew that without God's intervention in this whole situation, I could not get through it.

For six weeks I was in the hospital for induction chemotherapy, followed by outpatient cranial radiation, and then six more weeks of inpatient consolidation chemotherapy. I believe that God was in control of my situation the entire time. I saw His hand in my doctor's care and treatment plan. He was there when I received cards of encouragement from people I didn't even know. They had heard of my situation through friends and family members. He was there when the oncology nurses came into my room just to chat—especially when I was having a really tough day or was having trouble sleeping. He was there when my family would camp out in my room. Once I was in remission and discharged, I can remember how good it felt just to stand outside in the fresh air and look up at the trees.

Three-and-one-half years after being released from the hospital, the cancer came back! Guess what? God was still there! Sure, I was scared— perhaps even more than the first time around. Remembering that I had prayed for one more year, I thought I should be thankful that I had lived three times that long. Once again, during the treatment, I saw His hand in my situation. I have two siblings, one of whom was a perfect match for the bone marrow transplant I needed. I was blessed with the best doctor, the best nurses, the best friends, and a family that I wouldn't trade in for any other. I'm not trying to say the road was easy. It wasn't. But if God hadn't given up on me, then I wasn't giving up on me either!

It has been two-and-one-half years since I received my bone marrow transplant and almost seven years since I was first diagnosed with cancer. I'm feeling fine.

What has cancer brought me?

- A new best friend: my mom.
- A closeness to my dad that didn't exist before.
- A husband who has continued to stand by me through thick and thin.
- A membership in an elite group of individuals: Cancer Survivors!
- A chance to make a change in this world through helping others.
- A realization that miracles can even happen to me!

I'm not glad I was diagnosed with cancer. Yet, I can't imagine my life without all the positive things that have happened to me, including all the wonderful people I have met because of it.

Tammy M. Webster
Leukemia survivor, age 33
Ohio

The prayers of my family, friends, and church supported me with love and concern for months. At one time, my name was removed from the Pastor's prayer list. I felt as though I had been dropped on my head. It was really a tough week. I called and asked to be added back on the list. Many times, I have wanted to be of help to someone, feeling so inadequate when I said I would pray for them. Now, I realize that prayer makes a real difference.

Marilynne Dumers
Two-year breast cancer survivor
California

Now I can sit quietly in God's lap and be at peace, which I had not been able to do for more than 30 years.

Lora Wise McKenna
Cancer survivor
Pennsylvania

What Cancer Can't Do

Our greatest enemy is not disease, but despair.

One of the most dreaded sentences a patient may hear is "You have cancer." These words bring a chill to the heart. Although great progress has been made in treating cancer, recovery can be long and painful, and some people do not survive.

An enthusiastic believer in Christ, Dan Richardson lost his battle with cancer. But his life demonstrated that even though the physical body may be destroyed by disease, the spirit can remain triumphant. This poem was distributed at his memorial service.

> Cancer is so limited . . .
> It cannot cripple love
> It cannot shatter hope,
> It cannot erode faith,
> It cannot eat away peace
> It cannot destroy confidence,
> It cannot kill friendship
> It cannot shut out memories,
> It cannot silence courage
> It cannot invade the soul,
> It cannot reduce eternal life,
> It cannot quench the Spirit,
> It cannot lessen the power of the resurrection.

If an incurable disease has invaded your life, refuse to let it touch your spirit. Your body can be severely afflicted, and you may have a great struggle. But if you keep trusting God's love, your spirit will remain strong.

From **Our Daily Bread**

A Slow Fourth

When golf professional Paul Azinger learned in 1993 that he had cancer, he said, "I was in shock. I thought the doctor would tell me they had discovered some form of weird infection in my shoulder or possibly even a stress fracture. The one word I never expected to hear him say was *cancer*."

The good news was that it was curable. Now, after some time away from the professional golf tour for chemotherapy and radiation treatments, the man who's called "Zinger" is back, cancer-free.

When people ask Azinger if golf is still important to him, he says, "Yes and no. Yes, of course golf is important to me. I love the game; it is how I make a living. But no, golf is no longer at the top of my priority list. In fact, it runs a slow fourth. My priorities now are my God, my family, my friends, and golf. Golf is no longer my god. Golf is hitting a little white ball. God is my God, and God is a whole lot bigger than golf."

A serious disease has a way of putting things in perspective. First place belongs to the Lord: we are to worship nothing in our lives above Him. Make God number one in your life, and your dearest pastime on earth will become only a "slow fourth."

From "A Slow Fourth," by David C. Egner, **Our Daily Bread**
Copyright 1996 by RBC Ministries, Grand Rapids, MI.
Reprinted with permission.

The good Lord, a band of angels, my funny sense of humor, friends, and great family have helped me walk the road through my cancer experience.

Lori Walters
Six-year bone marrow transplant survivor and
10-year survivor of Hodgkin's disease
Pennsylvania

I Wear a Crown of Faith

Health is a crown on the head of the healthy.
Nobody feels it except the patient.

My name is Al-Muntaser Issa. I am 17 years old and from Jordan. I play the cello. Actually, it is difficult to pronounce my name correctly, so now I go by "Vic," which is the meaning of my native name.

I was diagnosed with cancer in Jordan. I immediately started a chemotherapy treatment course. After that, most of my doctors advised me to come to the United States. They had many reasons for this. Cancer treatment in the U.S. is more effective, my case was advanced, and the tumor had started in my left knee but cancer cells had spread to both of my lungs and one hip.

The most difficult thing for me was deciding about amputation surgery. The "mother" cell was in my knee and feeding the other cells. The doctors had to remove the tumor to control and kill the cancer that had spread to my hip and lungs. Although I was faced with this decision at the beginning of my diagnosis, I believed that I would not lose my leg. This belief made me strong physically and spiritually; however, I lost this hope when I ultimately had to make the decision to proceed with the surgery on May 23, 1996.

Actually, the amputation completely changed my way of thinking. I started to think about the British principle that states "Life over limb." To me, life no longer means physical life—I now believe in spiritual life. Many people seem to miss spiritual life these days. Now, while having this special opportunity to write, I still hold my beliefs and have faith in God. All that happens to human beings—good or bad—is a test. Those individuals who have a true belief in God should pass this test easily and wisely. Because of my belief, my ideas and principles about life made me happy, strong, and satisfied. Whatever happens in the future, I will face it with strength. I no longer care about limbs. Instead, I care about having a good brain and a strong heart that beats with feeling and love for all people and pumps the blood of faith. At last, I say, health is a crown on the head of the healthy. Nobody feels it except the patient.

Al-Muntaser "Vic" Issa
Young man receiving treatment for osteogenic sarcoma
Texas

Health is the crown that the well person wears and only the sick person sees. I was diagnosed and treated for ovarian cancer over a year ago. Now, each day that I feel well, I wear the crown, for health is now, and life is now. Life can change quickly, but today I wear the crown. I give thanks to God.

Dawn Stobbe
Ovarian cancer survivor
Nebraska

I did not fear. I did not worry. Whatever the outcome, I would be okay in God's hands. The transplant took place two months later. I was supported on a cushion of prayers offered by family, friends, and people I did not even know. I have learned to more fully and deeply appreciate the meaning and possibilities of my life.

Dorothy F. Reichenbach
Lymphoma survivor
Ohio

We are able to comfort, encourage, and experience each other in a unique way as we share our stories of God's presence in our lives. By the grace and love of God, I'm being empowered to live with more abandon, more joy, and more trust.

Elie Cole
Breast cancer survivor
Florida

My Friend Is a Hero

"God works all things together for good to those who love God, to those who are called according to his purpose" (Romans 8:28)

My friend Rhoda Simpson exemplifies my definition of a hero. This young woman has taken extremely adverse circumstances caused by cancer and turned them into a positive force that continues to motivate her. She embodies the scripture "God works all things together for good to those who love God, to those who are called according to his purpose" (Romans 8:28). It is her simple, childlike faith in God that sets her apart from others.

Rhoda's experiences with cancer began in October of 1993 when she went to the doctor for a "cold she couldn't shake." After several visits, the doctor discovered that Rhoda's real problem was in her abdomen. An ultrasound revealed a large pelvic mass. Rhoda was hospitalized the next day with difficulty breathing because a large tumor was pressing up on her diaphragm. Two days later, a 6.5-pound ovarian tumor was removed from the pelvis of this 110-pound, 16-year-old girl.

After the surgery, Rhoda required many transfusions due to bleeding. After recovering from anesthesia, Rhoda told her parents that she was "having difficulty focusing her eyes." The doctors waited a few days to see if her vision would improve after the medications wore off. She was taken to see an ophthalmologist. He discovered that Rhoda had bilateral central retinal arterial occlusions. Rhoda would never have central vision again—she would be almost totally blind, with only enough vision to count fingers from a distance of several feet. Rhoda was pronounced legally blind at age 16, with no hope of improvement.

The nurses and doctors at Carolinas Medical Center could not believe Rhoda's good spirits despite losing most of her vision and discovering that her tumor was a rare form of ovarian cancer. Rhoda would have to face three months of experimental chemotherapy. Her cheerful smile and winsome personality continued to win the hearts of every doctor and nurse on the unit.

Rhoda endured the chemotherapy with her usual joy and peace. She lost weight, all of her hair, and most of her energy, but she never lost her faith and hope in God. After Rhoda's first chemotherapy treatment, she sustained another terrible blow: Mary, her 18-year-old cousin, was killed in a car accident.

Rhoda finished high school with her graduating class—on time—with no central vision and only small "holes" of peripheral vision intact. She continued to be involved in church and school, singing and playing the piano in several choirs, working with preschool children at church, and writing for the school paper. Rhoda is a natural at counseling. She spent hours on the phone talking to the brokenhearted and discouraged, offering them the love and hope of God.

In the fall of 1995, Rhoda left home to begin her freshman year at Southeastern Christian College. She wanted to become a teacher of the visually impaired. To look at Rhoda, you would never know the hardships she has endured—surviving not only cancer, but blindness as well. Rhoda looks forward to student-teaching at a school for the blind in Florida. She hopes to motivate her students with her own hard-earned experiences with visual impairment. However, you cannot tell that she has any impairment at all. All you can see is a beautiful, vibrant, 19-year-old girl with a bright smile and an ever-positive outlook.

Sue Mehta, MSN, RN, OCN®, FNP
Oncology nurse
North Carolina

During the bone marrow transplant, when I received my own stem cells, I not only began to rebuild my cells, but my life as well. God gave me the wonderful opportunity to heal myself. He stood by me while I did.

Patricia L. Kinney
Breast cancer and bone marrow transplant survivor, a.k.a. "Alive and well!"
Arizona

The Bliss of Being

I began calling cancer my gift, my "God kiss."

We humans cherish many things. Perhaps more than anything we cherish life. Throughout 1994, I had a strong feeling that my life was drawing to a close. I experienced a certain sense. Voices spoke from within, and I recognized that I was being drawn by the One whom I fondly call "IS." I never spoke of these things. Only my journal reveals how much concern I dedicated to this undefined urgency of spirit.

On July 28, 1994, my doctor said, "Mrs. Konradi, it looks like you have cervical cancer and it appears to be well-developed." Three weeks and two surgeries later, another doctor spoke with my husband, Andy, and me in a hospital room. He said, "Lucy, your cancer is metastatic. We found tumors all the way into the periaortic area. The statistics for survival are not good. You probably have less than a 10% chance of surviving a year with this condition. We will do all that we can to help improve these statistics. Are you willing?"

I had no response to this question because my experiences as a recovering alcoholic told me that willingness happens in the *doing*. So, I knew I had to *do* the recommended program of treatment *to be* willing. At that moment—and ever since—I was filled with immense gratitude; however, I was not quite sure why I was so grateful. I became aware that gifts were being offered to me. Although I had always anticipated that such dire news would devastate every part of my being, I understood that my cancer was occurring for an unexplainable reason.

I sincerely felt blessed that I was given the knowledge that my life was drawing to a close. This knowledge provided me with time to prepare. I needed this time to understand grief from the vantage point of those who loved me and to sort through accumulations from years of living.

As the chemotherapy and radiation treatments

proceeded, my body rebelled with outrage in every cell. My spirit took flight into a new realm of being. I soon realized that I was seeing everything with a new vision. I had been transported into a state of peace. I began calling cancer my gift, my "God kiss," a confirmation of how much "IS" craved that I become part of Her/His Beingness. I have never felt victimized by cancer. This disease continues to be an immense, exquisite, beneficent, loving, and soul-expanding gift. My gratitude is unspeakable!

It is September 1996 as I write these words. I have had 18 chemotherapy treatments and seven weeks of daily radiation treatments. A few weeks ago, I heard the following words from my doctor: "Lucy, you are in remission." I think this means that I am supposed *to be* in a state of happiness because I am not going to die after all.

It is impossible to explain that cancer was the vehicle that God used to open an exquisite pathway for me to reach the Divine Presence. Cancer is the gift of a lifetime! I now clearly hear the words of the Divine Presence that tell me, "Among all things I create is you. You are unique and singular. There is not one other that is you. I love you for yourself alone. There is no earthly thought, word, or deed of yours that can ever separate us. Now you understand the *bliss of being*."

Lucy Martin Konradi
Two-year cervical cancer survivor
Texas

I was introduced to shelem, *a Hebrew word used in the time of Jesus to denote wholeness—a physical, emotional, and spiritual healing. God took my fear and doubt and turned what I thought would be a death sentence into life. We can survive and learn His lessons as we walk our individual path toward wholeness. I am learning to experience* shelem.

Marcey Corey
Celebrating three years as a
survivor of uterine cancer
Florida

All Through the Night

*Jesus sat by his bed and held his hand . . .
all through the night.*

Eight years ago, I had a bone marrow transplant for leukemia. When I went for my five-year checkup, the first person I tried to find was one of my favorite oncology nurses, Bill Cook, who had been particularly supportive during my ordeal. I was crushed to discover that Bill recently had died an untimely death.

When I first met Bill, I thought he looked familiar. My husband, Cal, also thought so. Then I suddenly realized where I had seen his face: Bill had a very strong resemblance to an image of Jesus Christ often seen in Sunday school classrooms. Cal agreed. Bill had a beard, shoulder-length brown hair, a peaceful countenance, and beautiful blue eyes that seemed to look deep into your soul.

I once sheepishly asked Bill, "Has anybody ever told you that you look like someone else?"

He replied, "Jesus Christ, right? One time a little boy who was staying at the hospital for a bone marrow transplant had his mother stay with him during the day. After a dinner break at home, she would return to his room and spend the night. Exhausted after several weeks of this, she accidentally fell asleep after dinner and didn't wake up until the next morning. Frantically, she dashed to the hospital, expecting to find a panicked child. 'Oh, Honey, I am so sorry!' she blurted out.

'That's okay, Mommy,' he replied. 'Jesus was here with me.'

'Sure he was, Darling,' she said, patting his hand.

'Look,' he interrupted. 'There he is now.'

"You should have seen the look on her face when she turned around and saw ME!" Bill recalled with a laugh.

Today, a teenage boy still remembers that long night far from home without his mother when "Jesus" sat by his bed and held his hand . . . all through the night.

Clare Buie Chaney, PhD
Licensed professional counselor and 10-year leukemia survivor
Texas

Never My Soul

Cancer, who are you?
I laugh in your face
and proclaim, "I am ME!"
For you will not steal my identity.

You invade my body, but never
my soul.
No matter your devastation,
I remain whole.
Whole to life and love and
laughter.

What are you after?
You vile disease!
I laugh in your face.
I do so with ease!

Carol Campbell
Wife, mother, and breast cancer survivor
Ohio

Surviving brings new challenges and
richness to life. I thank God for giving me
this day with the courage to live it to the
fullest.

Florence Langer
Survivor of recurrent breast cancer
Ohio

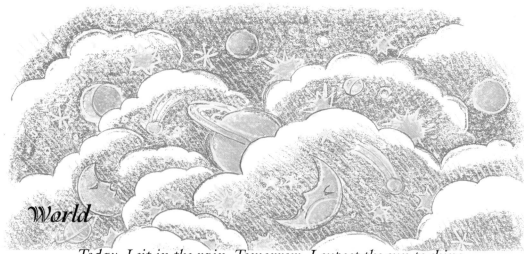

World

Today, I sit in the rain. Tomorrow, I expect the sun to shine.

It's amazing how your entire world can be turned upside down by a simple phone call. I always thought the worst day of my life was when I was first diagnosed with cancer. It was June 17, 1991. I found myself cast upon an adventure not of my choosing, but an adventure nonetheless. During my odyssey, I encountered many different experiences— some good, some not so good. I always felt that I needed to endure whatever hardships that were necessary to conquer the disease. I owed it to myself and to my family and friends to carry on.

An old Chinese proverb reads, "A journey of a thousand miles must begin with the first step." That first step is to seek proper medical attention. Early diagnosis and treatment are primary advantages in conquering cancer. But, cancer is not just a disease of the body. A person needs both emotional and mental support. The love and support of family and friends are key.

I don't know why I got my disease, but I do know that I am a better person today because of it. I am a better father, a better husband, and a better human being. During my first two years of treatment, I found myself in and out of several hospitals. Since then, for the past three years, I have done a lifetime of living!

I know what it means to face cancer and to battle it head-to-head. I know the physical part. I understand the emotional and mental part. My work this past year with people stricken with cancer has made my life very meaningful and filled with great purpose. Unfortunately, I have found that my journey is only partially over.

I always knew that my form of cancer had a high possibility of recurrence. I knew the doctors were testing me every 90 days for a reason. When the phone call came, however, I felt very small in a large world.

As I sat there alone, listening to the radio, I felt overcome with self-pity. Then a song called "World" by the pop group the Bee Gees came on, which I remembered from my teenage years. The first line is, "Now I've found that the world is round, and of course it rains every day." From those words, I regained my strength. I am not ready to quit. Recurrence is just another minor inconvenience. The world is round—and somewhere the sun is shining. Today, I sit in the rain. Tomorrow, I expect the sun to shine.

(My cancer appears to be in remission again, and I have not had chemotherapy since May 1996).

James W. Pleasant
Bone marrow transplant survivor
Ohio

In the big picture, we are but a heartbeat on a planet with billions. Don't tolerate small complaints such as the sun not coming out. Sometimes it is just hidden. Sometimes the love of God is hidden, too.

Brandon Creger
Osteosarcoma survivor
Michigan

Jeff never waited for a sunny day. His spirit, resolve, smile, friendliness, wit, determination, and attitude became a beacon of light to all who came in contact with him.

Tom Applegate
Father of Jeff Applegate,
who died at age 23 from malignant melanoma
Ohio

God, If You Call Me . . .

God, if You call me before I wake,
And I stand before your Heavenly Gate,
Do You mind if I come a little late?
I still have cookies to bake.

I am too young to be called.
I have young children who need me most of all.
They need me for all those things that only mothers can do,
Like wiping tears, and soothing fears, giving hugs, and collecting bugs.
God, what will they do?
I need them too.

I have a disease. Its name is cancer.
And every day I struggle for the answer.
You challenged me to fight,
So I fight with all my might.
I have the courage to live this life.

God, if I may be so bold.
Could I please grow old?
I have so much I need to do.
Could I please help my kids get through school?
What a full circle my life would be,
If I could just see my grandchildren grow to know me.

And while I'm asking, if it's not too much
Could I celebrate all the things in life
With the man I love so much?

God, if You call me, I love You so,
But I will fight it. I don't want to go.
God, call me when I am old and gray.
When I can no longer think or know the time of day.
That's the Day! I'll come right away.

So God, please wait for me, I have so much to do
And I'll gladly come when I am 92.

But if You call me—I will come.
But don't expect me to run.

Elaine Metzung
Mother of three young children and breast cancer survivor
Ohio

Out of pain arises incredible joy,
Wonder and awe—at the miracle of the
Everyday ordinariness of life—
I took so for granted before.

Betsy Firger
Attorney, wife, and mother of three teenagers and
four-year survivor of non-Hodgkin's lymphoma
Connecticut

One "feel-sorry-for-Juanita" night, I
was unable to reach three of my
friends by phone. So, I called God. I
told Him, "This is our battle, and You
and I are going to win it." I changed to
a healthy diet, began exercising, and
read everything I could get my
hands on about all kinds of cancer.
I became a volunteer for the
American Cancer Society. Over the past
six years, God has blessed me abundantly. I
am very happy. It is great to be alive.

Juanita Luster
Breast cancer survivor since October 1990
Missouri

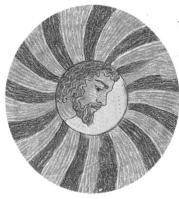

What's life all about? It's about:
fighting like hell,
bowing our heads and thanking God
for what we have,
experiencing hope, sadness, and
joy—all in one day.

Jennifer Gougas, RN, BSN, OCN®
Oncology nurse
California

These words provide spiritual strength for me:
"So do not fear, for I am with you;
do not be dismayed, for I am your God.
I will strengthen and help you;
I will uphold you with my righteous right
hand." (Isaiah 41:10)

Carolynn Sue Harrison
Wife, mother, and cancer survivor
Indiana

My cancer reinforced some of my deepest
values. It caused a powerful confirmation
of what really matters in life. Embrace life,
not death. The best way to live is to
appreciate all the miracles.

Florence Langer
Survivor of recurrent breast cancer
Ohio

My bone marrow transplant has been one of
the most challenging experiences I have ever
been through. Every morning that I wake
up and see the sun shining, I say a little
prayer to thank God for the extra day.

Shari R. Kahane, MD
Physician and survivor of breast cancer and bone marrow transplant
California

I never ask "Why?" or "Why me?" I can't see the whole picture. Only God sees that. I live one day at a time and thank God each day for His many blessings.

Gina Boyle
Bone marrow transplant recipient for acute lymphocytic leukemia in August 1996
Ohio

What lessons have I learned from these experiences? What have I yet to endure and face? Life seems so much more precious and fragile than it did before. The reality of my mortality has been brought home to me strongly. Cancer is best faced one day at a time. Worry and anxiety only serve to worsen the situation. Whether you have a long or short life expectancy, live whatever remains with the constant realization of what a great gift life really is. Treasure your loved ones and each moment that you spend with them.

Stanley F. Stefanski
Survivor of urinary and colon cancer
with liver metastasis
Illinois

Survival depends on your desire to live. Attitude is everything! I can't stress enough the importance of having strong, dependable people around you. Don't be afraid to ask for help when you need it . . . ASK!

Brandon Creger
Osteosarcoma survivor
Michigan

Author Index

Silver Linings: The Other Side of Cancer   235

Resources for Patients With Cancer

NATIONAL CANCER INSTITUTE-DESIGNATED COMPREHENSIVE CANCER CENTERS

Cancer Center of Wake Forest University at the Bowman Gray School of Medicine
Medical Center Boulevard
Winston-Salem, NC 27157
919-748-4354

Columbia University Comprehensive Cancer Center
College of Physicians and Surgeons
630 W. 168th Street
New York, NY 10032
212-305-6905

Dana-Farber Cancer Institute
44 Binney Street
Boston, MA 02115
617-632-3000

Duke Comprehensive Cancer Center
P.O. Box 3814
Durham, NC 27710
919-684-5810

Fox Chase Cancer Center
7701 Burholme Avenue
Philadelphia, PA 19111
215-728-2570

Fred Hutchinson Cancer Research Center
1124 Columbia Street
Seattle, WA 98104
206-667-5000

James Cancer Hospital and Research Institute
410 W. 10th Avenue
Columbus, OH 43210
614-293-8619

The Johns Hopkins Oncology Center
600 N, Wolfe Street
Baltimore, MD 21205
410-955-8638

Jonsson Comprehensive Cancer Center
University of California at Los Angeles
10833 LeConte Avenue
Los Angeles, CA 90024
310-825-5268

Kaplan Cancer Center
New York University Medical Center
462 First Avenue
New York, NY 10016
212-263-6485

The Kenneth T. Norris, Jr. Comprehensive Cancer Center
University of Southern California
1441 Eastlake Avenue
Los Angeles, CA 90033
213-226-2370

Lombardi Cancer Research Center
Georgetown University Medical Center
3800 Reservoir Road NW
Washington, DC 20007
202-687-2192

Mayo Comprehensive Cancer Center
200 First Street SW
Rochester, MN 55905
507-284-3413

Memorial Sloan-Kettering Cancer Center
1275 York Avenue
New York, NY 10021
800-525-2225

Meyer L. Prentis Comprehensive Cancer Center of Metropolitan Detroit
110 E Warren Avenue
Detroit, MI 48201
313-745-4329

Norris Cotton Cancer Center Dartmouth-Hitchcock Medical Center
1 Medical Center Drive
Lebanon, NH 03756
603-650-5527

Pittsburgh Cancer Institute
200 Meyran Avenue
Pittsburgh, PA 15213
800-537-4063

Roswell Park Cancer Institute
Elm and Carlton Streets
Buffalo, NY 14263
800-767-9355

Sylvester Comprehensive Cancer Center
University of Miami Medical School
1475 NW 12th Avenue
Miami, FL 33136
305-545-1000

University of Alabama at Birmingham Comprehensive Cancer Center
1824 Sixth Avenue S
Birmingham, AL 35294
205-934-5077

University of Arizona Cancer Center
1501 N. Campbell Avenue
Tucson, AZ 85724
602-626-6372

University of Michigan Comprehensive Cancer Center
101 Simpson Drive
Ann Arbor, MI 48109
313-936-9583

University of North Carolina Lineberger Comprehensive Cancer Center
University of North Carolina School of Medicine
Chapel Hill, NC 27599
919-966-3036

University of Pennsylvania Cancer Center
Penn Tower Hotel, 6th Floor
3400 Spruce Street
Philadelphia, PA 19104
215-662-6364

The University of Texas M.D. Anderson Cancer Center
1515 Holcombe Boulevard
Houston, TX 77030
713-792-3245

Vermont Cancer Center
University of Vermont
1 S. Prospect Street
Burlington, VT 05401
802-656-4414

Wisconsin Clinical Cancer Center
University of Wisconsin
600 Highland Avenue
Madison, WI 53792
608-263-8600

Yale University Comprehensive
Cancer Center
P.O. Box 3333, LEPH-139
New Haven, CT 06510
203-785-6338

HOSPITALS WITH MULTIDISCIPLINARY SECOND-OPINION CLINICS

Arizona Cancer Center
Tucson, AZ
602-626-2900

Cedars Medical Center
Miami, FL
305-325-5691

City of Hope National Medical Center
Duarte, CA
818-359-8111

Cleveland Clinic Cancer Center
Cleveland, OH
216-444-2444

DeKalb Medical Center
Atlanta-Decatur, GA
404-501-5559

Ireland Cancer Center
Cleveland, OH
216-844-5432

Loyola University Medical Center
Chicago, IL
708-216-3336

Meyer L. Prentis Comprehensive Cancer Center of Metropolitan Detroit
Detroit, MI
313-993-0335

Montefiore Medical Center
Bronx, NY
212-920-4826

Mount Sinai Cancer Center
New York, NY
212-241-6361

Northwestern University
Chicago, IL
312-908-5284

Regional Cancer Center Lourdes
Binghamton, NY
607-798-5431

Regional Cancer Foundation
San Francisco, CA
415-775-9956

St. Jude Children's Research Hospital
Memphis, TN
901-522-0301

St. Vincent Cancer Center
Little Rock, AR
501-660-3900

Thompson Cancer Survival Center
Knoxville, TN
615-541-1757

University of California at San Diego Cancer Center
San Diego, CA
619-543-3456

University of Colorado Cancer Center
Denver, CO
303-372-1550

University of Iowa Cancer Center
Iowa City, IA
319-356-3584

University of Rochester Cancer Center
Rochester, NY
716-275-4911

UTMB Cancer Center
Galveston, TX
409-772-1164

INFORMATION, SERVICES, AND SUPPORT FOR PATIENTS WITH CANCER

Air Life Line
1716 X Street
Sacramento, CA 95818
916-446-0995
800-446-1231

American Brain Tumor Association (ABTA)
2720 River Road
Suite 146
Des Plaines, IL 60018
847-827-9910
800-886-2282 (patient line)
E-mail: ABTA@aol.com

American Cancer Society (ACS)
1599 Clifton Road, NE
Atlanta, GA 30329-4251
404-320-3333 (general info)
404-329-7623 (patient services)
800-ACS-2345 (for cancer info)
Web site: http://www.cancer.org

American Institute for Cancer Research (AICR)
1759 R Street, NW
Washington, DC 20069
202-328-7744 (general information)
800-843-8114 (Nutrition Hotline, publications department)

American Lung Association
1740 Broadway
New York, NY 10019-4374
212-315-8700

American Medical Support Flight Team (Angel Flight)
3237 Donald Douglas Loop S
Santa Monica, CA 90405
310-390-2958
310-456-2035 (24-hour hotline)

American Red Cross
431 18th Street NW
Washington, DC 20006
202-737-8300

Bone Marrow Transplant Family Support Network
P.O. Box 845
Avon, CT 06001
800-826-9376

Breast Cancer Information Clearinghouse
Web site:
http://www.nysernet.org/bcic/

Canadian Cancer Society
Web site:
http://www.ncf.carleton.ca:
12345.freeport/health/ccs/menu

Cancer Guidance Hotline
1323 Forbes Avenue, Suite 200
Pittsburgh, PA 15239
412-261-2211

Cancer Support Network
802 E. Jetterson
Bloomington, IL 61701
309-829-2273

CanSurmount
(contact local ACS office)

Center for Attitudinal Healing
19 Main Street
Tiburon, CA 94920
415-435-5022

Center for Medical Consumers
237 Thompson Street
New York, NY 10012
212-674-7105

Children's Oncology Camps of America
75 Richland Memorial Park
Suite 203
Columbia, SC 29203
803-434-3533

Children's Oncology Camps of America
2309 W Whiteoaks Drive
Suite B
Springfield, IL 62704
217-793-3949

Choice In Dying (CID)
200 Varick Street, 10th Floor
New York, NY 10014-4810
212-366-5540
or 800-989-WILL (9455)
E-mail: cid@choices.org
Web site: http://www.choices.org

Consumer Health Information Research Institute
3521 Broadway
Kansas City, MO 64111
800-821-6671

Encore^plus
YWCA of the USA Encore^plus Program
(breast and cervical cancer)
Office of Women's Health Initiatives
624 9th Street, NW, 3rd Floor
Washington, DC 20001
202-628-3636/800-95-EPLUS

Food and Drug Administration
Office of Consumer Affairs,
HFE-88
5600 Fishers Lane
Rockville, MD 20857
800-532-4440

I Can Cope
(contact a local ACS office)

International Association of Laryngectomees
404-329-7561
404-329-7622

International Pain Foundation
909 NE 43rd Street, Suite 306
Seattle, WA 98105
206-547-2157

Leukemia Society of America, Inc.
600 Third Avenue
New York, NY 10016
212-573-8484
800-955-4LSA (information hotline)

Look Good, Feel Better (LGFB)
The Cosmetic, Toiletry, and Fragrance Association Foundation
1101 17th Street NW
Suite 300
Washington, DC 20036
202-331-1770
800-395-LOOK

Lymphoma Research Foundation of America
8800 Venice Bouevard, #207
Los Angeles, CA 90034
310-204-7040

Make-A-Wish Foundation of America
100 West Clarendon, Suite 2200
Phoenix, AZ 85013-3518
800-722-WISH
or 602-279-WISH

Man to Man
(prostate cancer)
910 Contento Street
Sarasota, FL 34242
813-349-1719
813-355-4987

National Alliance of Breast Cancer Organizations (NABCO)
9 East 37th Street, 10th Floor
New York, NY 10016
800-719-9154
Web site: http://www.nabco.org

National Association of Hospital Hospitality Houses, Inc.
4013 West Jackson Street
Muncie, IN 47304
800-542-9730

National Bone Marrow Donor Program
3433 Broadway Street NE
Suite 400
Minneapolis, MN 55413
800-654-1247 (hotline/donors)
800-526-7809 (general business and recipients)

National Cancer Care Foundation, Cancer Care, Inc.
1180 Avenue of the Americas
New York, NY 10036
800-813-HOPE
212-302-2400
Web site:
http://www.cancercareinc.org/

National Cancer Institute (NCI)
Cancer Information Service (CIS)
31 Center Drive MSC2580
Building 31, Room 10A07
Bethesda, MD 20892-2580
800-4-CANCER
or 800-422-6237
800-332-8615 (TTY)
301-496-5583
NCI Cancer Net:
http://wwwicic.nci.nih.gov
NCI Cancer Kids Page:
http://wwwicic.nci.nih.gov/occdocs/KidsHome.html

National Coalition for Cancer Survivorship (NCCS)
1010 Wayne Avenue, Suite 505
Silver Spring, MD 20910
301-650-8868

National Council Against Health Fraud Resource Center
3521 Broadway
Kansas City, MO 64111
800-821-6671

National Family Caregivers Association
9621 East Bexhill Drive
Kensington, MD 20895
800-896-3650

National Health Information Center
P.O. Box 1133
Washington, DC 20013
301-565-4167 (Maryland)
800-336-4797

National Leukemia Association, Inc.
585 Stewart Avenue, Suite 536
Garden City, NY 11530
516-222-1944

National Lymphedema Network (NLN)
2211 Post Street, Suite 404
San Francisco, CA 94115
800-541-3259 (hotline)
E-mail: lymphnet@hooked.net
Web site: http://www.hooked.net/~lymphnet

National Women's Health Network
514 10th Street NW, Suite 400
Washington, DC 20004
202-347-1140

Ostomy Rehabilitation Program
(contact a local ACS office)

Prostate Health Program of New York
785 Park Avenue
New York, NY 10021
212-988-8888

R.A. Bloch Cancer Foundation, Inc.
The Cancer Hotline
4410 Main Street
Kansas City, MO 64111
816-932-8453

Reach to Recovery Program
(contact a local ACS office)

Ronald McDonald Houses
Ronald McDonald House Charities
One Kroc Drive
Oak Brook, IL 60521
708-575-7070

Share
(support for breast and cervical cancer)
19 W 44th Street, Suite 415
New York, NY 10036
212-382-2111

The Skin Cancer Foundation
245 Fifth Avenue, Suite 2402
New York, NY 10016
212-725-5176

United Cancer Council, Inc.
1803 N Meridian Street
Indianapolis, IN 46202
317-923-6490

United Ostomy Association, Inc.
36 Executive Park, Suite 120
Irvine, CA 92714
714-660-8624
800-826-0826

Wellness Community National Headquarters
2200 Colorado Avenue
Santa Monica, CA 90404
310-453-2300

Y-ME National Breast Cancer Organization
212 W. Van Buren, 5th Floor
Chicago, IL 60607-3908
800-986-9505 (Hispanic hotline)
312-986-8228 (24-hour hotline)
800-221-2141 (toll-free hotline, 24 hours)

Y-ME Breast Cancer Support Program, Inc.
18220 Harwood Avenue
Homewood, IL 60430
708-799-8228 (24-hour hotline)
800-221-2141

RESOURCES

American Foundation for Urologic Disease, Inc.
300 West Pratt Street, Suite 401
Baltimore, MD 21201-2463
410-727-2908
E-mail: admin@afud.org

Bone Marrow Transplant (BMT) Newsletter
1985 Spruce Avenue
Highland Park, IL 60035
708-831-1913

Cancer Federation, Inc.
711 West Ramsey
P.O. Box 1298
Banning, CA 92220
909-849-HEAL

Cancer Communication
Patient Advocates for Advanced Cancer Treatment (PAACT)
1143 Parmelee NW
Grand Rapids, MI 49504
616-453-1477
616-453-1351 (information available on voicemail)

Cancer-FAQ
A current list of oncology/cancer services can be reached on the Internet through the home page of Medicine On Line. The URL is http://www.meds.com/.

Cancer Research Institute
681 Fifth Avenue
New York, NY 10022
212-688-7515
800-992-2623

Cancer Support Network
Esse House, Suite L10
Baum Boulevard at South Negley Avenue

Pittsburgh, PA 15206
412-361-8600

CancerNet™
NCI International Cancer Information Center
9030 Old Georgetown Road
Bethesda, MD 20814-1519
800-NCI-7890
Web site: http://cancernet.nci.nih.gov/

Cancervive
6500 Wilshire Boulevard
Suite 500
Los Angeles, CA 90048
310-203-9232

Candlelighters
7910 Woodmont Avenue
Suite 460
Bethesda, MD 20814
301-657-8401 (Maryland)
800-366-2223

The Chemotherapy Foundation
183 Madison Avenue, Suite 403
New York, NY 10016
212-213-9292

CONVERSATIONS! The Newsletter for Women Who Are Fighting Ovarian Cancer
P.O. Box 7948
Amarillo, TX 79114-7948
806-355-2656.

Coping
Media America, Inc.
P.O. Box 682268
Franklin, TN 37068-2268
615-790-2400
e-mail: Copingmag@aol.com

Corporate Angel Network (CAN)
Westchester County Airport
Building 1
White Plains, NY 10604
914-328-1313

Families Against Cancer (FACT)
P.O. Box 588
DeWitt, NY 13214
315-446-6385

Gynecologic Cancer Foundation
401 North Michigan Avenue
Chicago, IL 60611
312-644-6610

International Myeloma Foundation
2120 Stanley Hills Drive
Los Angeles, CA 90046
800-452-CURE

Living Through Cancer
323 Eighth Street SW
Albuquerque, NM 87102
505-242-3263

LymphEdema Foundation
P.O. Box 834
San Diego, CA 92014-0834
800-LYMPH-DX
or 800-596-7439

Lymphoma Research Foundation of America, Inc.
2318 Prosser Avenue
Los Angeles, CA 90064
310-470-4912

Make Today Count
1235 East Cherokee
Springfield, MO 65804-2263
417-885-2273
800-432-2273

Nabco News
National Association of Breast Cancer Organizations
2280 Avenue of the Americas
New York, NY 10036
212-719-0154

National Black Leadership Initiative on Cancer (NBLIC)
6130 Executive Boulevard (EPN 240)
Bethesda, MD 20892
301-496-8589

National Bone Marrow Transplant Link (BMT Link)
29209 Northwestern Highway, #624
Southfield, MI 48034
800-LINK-BMT

National Breast Cancer Coalition
1707 L Street NW, Suite 1060
Washington, DC 20036
202-265-6854

National Cancer Survivors Day (NCSD) Foundation, Inc.
P.O. Box 682285
Franklin, TN 37068-2285
615-794-3006

National Coalition for Cancer Research (NCCR)
Capitol Associates Inc.
426 C Street NE
Washington, DC 20002
202-544-1880

National Hispanic Leadership Initiative on Cancer
En Accion Coordinating Center
South Texas Health Research Center
The University of Texas Health Sciences Center at San Antonio
7703 Floyd Curl Drive
San Antonio, TX 78284-7791
Amelie G. Ramirez, DrPH
Principal Investigator
210-614-4496

National Marrow Donor Program (NMDP)
Coordinating Center
3433 Broadway Street NE
Suite 500
Minneapolis, MN 55413
800-526-7809
800-627-7692
or 800-MARROW-2
Web site: http://www.marrow.org

National Surgical Adjuvant Breast and Bowel Projects (NSABP)
Operations Center
230 McKee Place, Suite 402
Pittsburgh, PA 15213
412-383-1400

NCCS Networker
National Coalition for Cancer Survivorship
1010 Wayne Avenue
Silver Spring, MD 20910
301-650-8868

SEARCH
National Brain Tumor Foundation (NBTF)
785 Market Street, Suite 1600
San Francisco, CA 94103
415-284-0208
800-934-CURE

Support for People With Oral and Head and Neck Cancer, Inc.
P.O. Box 53
Locust Valley, NY 11560
516-759-5333

Surviving!
Stanford University Medical Center
Patient Research Center
Room H0103
Division of Radiation Oncology
300 Pasteur Drive
Stanford, CA 94305
415-723-7881

Susan G. Komen Breast Cancer Foundation
5005 LBJ Freeway
Suite 370
Dallas, TX 75244
214-450-1777
800-I'M AWARE
or 800-462-9273 (national helpline)

United Ostomy Association (UOA)
36 Executive Park
Suite 120
Irvine, CA 92714
714-660-8624
800-826-0826

PEDIATRICS

Association for Research of Childhood Cancer
P.O. Box 251
Buffalo, NY 14225-0251
716-689-8922

Association for the Care of Children's Health (ACCH)
7910 Woodmont Avenue
Suite 300
Bethesda, MD 20814
301-654-6549

Federation for Children With Special Needs
617-482-2915

National Childhood Cancer Foundation
800-458-6223
Web site: http://www.nccf.org/

SKIP (Sick Kids Need Involved People)
212-421-9160

We Care Foundation/Camp Dream Street
P.O. Box 3431
Fort Smith, AR 72913
501-441-6292

PROFESSIONAL ORGANIZATIONS/ RESOURCES

Agency for Health Care Policy and Research (AHCPR)
AHCPR Publication Clearinghouse
P.O. Box 8547
Silver Spring, MD 20907
800-358-9295

American Academy of Hospice and Palliative Medicine
P.O. Box 14288
Gainesville, FL 32604-2288
352-377-8900

American Association for Cancer Education (AACE)
University of Texas
M.D. Anderson Cancer Center-189
1515 Holcombe Boulevard
Houston, TX 77030
713-792-3020

American Association for Cancer Research
Public Leger Building, Suite 816
150 South Independence Mall West
Philadelphia, PA 19106-3483
215-440-9300

American College of Oncology Administrators
30555 Southfield Road
Suite 150
Southfield, MI 48076
810-540-4310

American College of Radiology
1891 Preston White Drive
Reston, VA 22091

American Pain Society
708-375-4715

American Society for Therapeutic Radiology and Oncology
1891 Preston White Drive
Reston, VA 20191
800-962-7876; 703-716-7588

American Society of Clinical Oncology
435 North Michigan Avenue
Suite 1717
Chicago, IL 60611
312-644-0828

American Society of Pain Management Nurses (ASPMN)
1550 South Coast Highway
Suite 201
Laguna Beach, CA 92651
714-545-1305

American Society of Plastic and Reconstructive Surgeons
444 East Algonquin Road
Arlington Heights, IL 60005
312-228-9900
800-635-0635 (recorded referral message)

Association of Community Cancer Centers (ACCC)
11600 Nebel Street
Suite 201
Rockville, MD 20852
301-984-9496

Association of Nurses in AIDS Care (ANAC)
1555 Connecticut Avenue, NW
Suite 200
Washington, DC 20036
202-462-1038
E-mail: AIDSnurses@aol.com

Association of Oncology Social Work (AOSW)
1910 E. Jefferson Street
Baltimore, MD 21205
410-614-3990

Association of Pediatric Oncology Nurses (APON)
4700 West Lake Avenue
Glenview, IL 60025-1485
847-375-4724

Centers for Disease Control
Web site: http://www.cdc.gov/cdc.htm

Hospice Nurses Association (HNA)
5512 Northumberland Street
Pittsburgh, PA 15217-1131
412-687-3231

International Society of Nurses in Cancer Care
The Royal College of Nursing
20 Cavendish Square
London W1M 0AB
071-495-6119

Intravenous Nurses Society (INS)
Fresh Pond Square
10 Fawcett Street

Cambridge, MA 02138
617-441-3008

League of Intravenous Therapy Education (LITE)
P.O. Box 3102
McKeesport, PA 15134-3102
412-678-5025

National Association of Physicians for the Environment
6401 Rockledge Drive
Suite 412
Bethesda, MD 20817
301-571-9791

National Foundation for Cancer Research (NFCR)
800-321-CURE (free information)

National Kidney Cancer Association
1234 Sherman Avenue
Suite 200
Evanston, IL 60202
708-332-1051

Oncology Nursing Society
501 Holiday Drive
Pittsburgh, PA 15220-2749
412-921-7373

Resource Center for State Cancer Pain Initiatives
3671 Medical Sciences Center
1300 University Avenue
Madison, WI 53706
608-265-4013

Society for Biological Therapy (SBT)
P.O. Box 5630
Madison, WI 53705-0630
608-276-6640

Society of Gynecologic Oncologists
401 North Michigan Avenue
Chicago, IL 60611
312-644-6610
E-mail: Sgo@Sba.com
Web site: http://www.sgo.org

Society of Surgical Oncology
85 W. Algonquin Road, #550
Arlington Heights, IL 60005
708-427-1400

PUBLIC GENERAL INFORMATION

CancerFax®
National Cancer Institute (NCI)
International Cancer Information Center
9030 Old Georgetown Road
Bethesda, MD 20814-1519
301-402-5874 (on fax machine handset)
800-624-7890 (for technical assistance)

Combined Health Information Database (CHID)
National Institutes of Health
Box CHID
9000 Rockville Pike
Rockville, MD 20892

Head and Neck Cancer Information Service
Rush Cancer Institute
Rush-Presbyterian-St. Luke's Medical Center
1725 West Harrison Street, Suite 863
Chicago, IL 60612
312-563-2322

The (Mary-Helen) Mautner Project for Lesbians With Cancer
1707 L Street, NW, Suite 1060
Washington, DC 20036
202-332-5536 (voice/TTY)

National Cancer Institute (NCI) Information Associates Program
9030 Old Georgetown Road
Bethesda, MD 20814-1519
800-NCI-7890 (U.S.)
301-496-7600 (international)

Office of Minority Health Resource Center (OMH-RC)
U.S. Department of Health and Human Services
P.O. Box 37337
Washington, DC 20013-7337
800-444-6472

U.S. Department of Labor Occupational Safety and Health Administration (OSHA)
Directorate of Technical Support
200 Constitution Avenue, NW
Washington, DC 20210
202-219-7047

PATIENT INFORMATION & SUPPORT SERVICES

Alliance of Lung Cancer Advocacy, Support, and Education, and Spirit and Breath
800-298-2436

Cancer Information and Support
800-221-2141

The Compassionate Friends
708-990-0010

Feminine Image
800-730-1123

Gilda's Club
212-647-9700

International Association of Cancer Victors and Friends, Inc.
310-822-5032

International Myeloma Foundation
800-452-CURE

Johanna's On Call to Mend Esteem, Inc.
518-482-4178

The Mathews Foundation for Prostate Cancer Research
800-234-6284

National Association for Continence (NAFC)
864-579-7900
800-BLADDER
AMC Cancer Research Center
800-525-3777
303-233-6501 (in CO)

National Kidney Cancer Association
708-332-1051

National Consumer Insurance Helpline
800-942-4242

National Self-Help Clearinghouse
212-642-2944

PDQ (Physician Data Query)
800-4-CANCER

Pharmaceutical Research and Manufacturers of America
800-PMA-INFO

Prostate Cancer Services Network
800-828-7866

U.S. Library of Medicine
Web site: http://www.ntm.nih.gov/

World Health Organization
Web site: http://www.who.ch/

Silver Linings
The Other Side of Cancer

This unique book shares the insights and comforting words of people who have experienced cancer -- either as a patient, family member, friend or healthcare professional. Their stories describe lessons that helped them find new perspectives on life.

These stories were written by people from all walks of life, demonstrating that cancer shows no respect for age, gender, social class or race. They tell of love and laughter, family and friends, miracles, triumphs, and an appreciation of everyday life.

The people in these stories discovered a strength and courage they never knew they had -- before their lives were touched by cancer. Their words will touch your heart and rekindle your spirit for life. To order, please return the form at the right, or contact an ONS customer service representative at 412-921-7373.

Silver Linings: The Other Side of Cancer
Edited by Shirley M. Gullo, RN, MSN, OCN®
and Elaine Glass, RN, MS, OCN®

Silver Linings: The Other Side of Cancer
Order Form

A check (made payable to the Oncology Nursing Press, Inc.) or credit card information must accompany your order.

Before May 15, 1997: ONS members - $11.60   Non-members - $15.60

After May 15, 1997: ONS members - $14.50   Non-members - $19.50

❏ Check ❏ Visa ❏ Master Card   ONS Member ID # _____

Credit Card # _____

Exp. _____ Signature _____

Name _____

Address _____

_____

Daytime Phone # _____

Silver

Item #	Qty.	Price	Total
BKSL9701			

Shipping and Handling Charges
Within the US:
Orders up to $25 $5
25.01 to $50 $6
50.01 to $100 $7
Over $100   7% of total purchase price
Outside US: 40% of total purchase price

PA residents must include 7% sales tax

Type of Shipping
(see below)
Shipping Charges

TOTAL

There is a 20% discount on a purchase of ten or more copies of the same item.

Allow 2-3 weeks for delivery. Orders within the US will be shipped UPS Ground (unless otherwise specified). Orders outside the US will be shipped USPS Express Mail International. Next Day Air Service is available at actual cost (you will be charged/invoiced). If actual shipping cost exceeds amounts shown here, you may be charged the difference.

Mail your order to: Oncology Nursing Press, Inc. -- Department 8847, Pittsburgh, PA 15278-8847
or Fax to: 412-921-6565

About the Editors

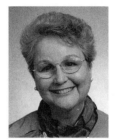

Shirley M. Gullo, RN, MSN, OCN®, is an oncology clinical nurse specialist at the Cleveland Clinic Cancer Center, where she has worked with patients with cancer and their families for 25 years. She is a nationally known speaker and has published numerous articles. As a charter member of the Oncology Nursing Society (ONS), she has served in many roles within the organization since 1975. She is married to Joseph Gullo, and together they have raised seven children. Shirley and her husband reside in Chesterland, OH.

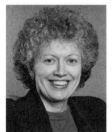

Elaine Glass, RN, MS, OCN®, has been an oncology nurse in both clinical and management roles for 25 years at the Ohio State University Medical Center/The James Cancer Hospital and Research Institute. She currently is the clinical nurse specialist in their newly developed palliative medicine–hospice program. She has been a very active member of ONS since 1977, when she first attended the ONS Congress and met a new friend, Shirley Gullo. Elaine is known for her smile, sense of humor, and collection of frogs, cartoons, and inspirational quotes. She resides in Columbus, OH, with her husband, Steve, and their beagle mix, Ollie.

About the Illustrator

Maria Gamiere has been illustrating greeting cards and related products for American Greetings Corporation for the past 34 years, first on the staff as a designer and, after the birth of her children, as a freelancer, working from her home in South Euclid, OH, where she still resides with her husband and one of their two sons.